G.MUSTAFA SOOMRO

Essential Guide to Generic Skills

B.MUSTAFA SOOMRO

Essential Guide to Generic Skills

Nicola Cooper
Specialist Registrar in General Internal Medicine and Care of the Elderly
Yorkshire, UK

Kirsty Forrest
Consultant in Anaesthesia
The Leeds Teaching Hospitals NHS Trust Leeds, UK

Paul Cramp
Consultant in Anaesthesia and Intensive Care
Bradford Teaching Hospitals NHS Trust Bradford, UK

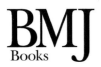

Blackwell
Publishing

© 2006 Nicola Cooper, Kirsty Forrest and Paul Cramp
Published by Blackwell Publishing Ltd
BMJ Books is an imprint of the BMJ Publishing Group Limited, used under licence

Blackwell Publishing, Inc., 350 Main Street, Malden, Massachusetts 02148-5020, USA
Blackwell Publishing Ltd, 9600 Garsington Road, Oxford OX4 2DQ, UK
Blackwell Publishing Asia Pty Ltd, 550 Swanston Street, Carlton, Victoria 3053, Australia

The right of the Author to be identified as the Author of this Work has been asserted in
accordance with the Copyright, Designs and Patents Act 1988.

All rights reserved. No part of this publication may be reproduced, stored in a retrieval
system, or transmitted, in any form or by any means, electronic, mechanical,
photocopying, recording or otherwise, except as permitted by the UK Copyright,
Designs and Patents Act 1988, without the prior permission of the publisher.

First published 2006

1 2006

Library of Congress Cataloging-in-Publication Data

Cooper, Nicola.
   Essential guide to generic skills / Nicola Cooper, Kirsty Forrest,
Paul Cramp.
      p. ; cm.
   Includes bibliographical references and index.
   ISBN-13: 978-1-4051-3973-1 (pbk. : alk. paper)
   ISBN-10: 1-4051-3973-0 (pbk. : alk.paper)
1. Medical care—Great Britain. 2. Clinical competence—Great
Britain. I. Forrest, Kirsty. II. Cramp, Paul. III. Title.
   [DNLM: 1. Medicine—Great Britain. 2. Ethics, Medical—Great
Britain. 3. Medical Errors—Great Britain. 4. Professional
Competence—Great Britain. 5. Professional Practice—Great Britain. W
21 C777e 2006]

RA418.3.G7C66 2006
362.10941—dc22

                                                            2006016790

ISBN-10: 1-4051-3973-0
ISBN-13: 978-1-4051-3973-1

A catalogue record for this title is available from the British Library

Set by Charon Tec Ltd, Chennai, India, www.charontec.com
Printed and bound by Replika Press Pvt. Ltd, Haryana, India

Commissioning Editor: Mary Banks
Editorial Assistant: Vicky Pittman
Development Editors: Vicki Donald and Simone Dudziak
Production Controller: Debbie Wyer
Illustrations by Hayley Oakes, www.hayleyoakes.co.uk

For further information on Blackwell Publishing, visit our website:
www.blackwellpublishing.com

The publisher's policy is to use permanent paper from mills that operate a sustainable
forestry policy, and which has been manufactured from pulp processed using acid-free
and elementary chlorine-free practices. Furthermore, the publisher ensures that the text
paper and cover board used have met acceptable environmental accreditation standards.

Blackwell Publishing makes no representation, express or implied, that the drug dosages in
this book are correct. Readers must therefore always check that any product mentioned in
this publication is used in accordance with the prescribing information prepared by the
manufacturers. The author and the publishers do not accept responsibility or legal liability
for any errors in the text or for the misuse or misapplication of material in this book.

Contents

List of contributors

Professionalism
Patsy Stark, Senior Lecturer in Medical Education, Academic Unit of Medical Education, Sheffield University, Sheffield

The consultation
Kay Brennan, Registrar in General Practice, Yorkshire

The Mental Health Act and common law
Rob Waller, Lecturer in Psychiatry, University of Leeds, Leeds

Adult and child protection
Rosemary Young, Social Worker (Care of the Elderly), Leeds General Infirmary, Leeds
Gillian Fox, Specialist Registrar in General Internal Medicine and Care of the Elderly, Yorkshire
Jonathan Garside, Consultant Paediatrician, Huddersfield Royal Infirmary, Huddersfield

Ethical principles in healthcare
Bruno Rushworth, Registrar in General Practice, Yorkshire

Advance directives
Susan McLaughlin, Senior House Officer in General Internal Medicine, Leeds General Infirmary, Leeds

End of life issues
Dominic Bell, Consultant in Intensive Care Medicine, Leeds General Infirmary, Leeds

Infection control
Philip Stanley, Consultant in Infectious Diseases, Director of Infection Prevention and Control, Bradford Teaching Hospitals, Bradford

Teaching small groups
Harry Walmsley, Consultant Anaesthetist, East Sussex Hospitals NHS Trust, Sussex
Michael Clapham, Consultant in Intensive Care Medicine and Anaesthesia, University Hospital, Birmingham Foundation NHS Trust, Birmingham

Teaching a skill
Dave Murray, Consultant Anaesthetist, James Cook University Hospital, Middlesborough

How doctors are assessed
Julian Archer, Medical Education Research Fellow for the Foundation Assessment Programme and Specialist Registrar in Paediatrics, Sheffield University, Sheffield

Foreword

It gives me great pleasure to write the foreword for this excellent book. It has been produced because the Foundation Programme Curriculum expects doctors in the first 2 years after qualification (Foundation Years) to become skilled in the care of the acutely ill and also in the generic skills that will help all graduates to become better doctors. Up until now, these skills have always been an implied sub-plot in other curricula. There are now explicitly stated competences that need to be acquired in these generic areas, all of which are covered in this book.

This excellent monograph makes easy reading and the recommendation at the beginning to dip in and out of it, is absolutely right. It will help planners of Foundation Programme education sessions to devise meaningful and interesting sessions and, most importantly, it will help under-graduates and foundation trainees to understand the importance of generic skills in clinical practice.

The layout is particularly attractive and easy to read and I would commend the little clinical scenarios as fun to do.

The production of this book and the content thereof brings to life the Foundation Curriculum in a way that doctors at all levels of training will find interesting and appropriate. Their educational supervisors may also find individual parts of it particularly attractive.

Ed Neville MD, FRCP
Chair, Foundation Programme Committee
Academy of Medical Royal Colleges

Introduction

The UK Foundation Programme Curriculum has two main themes: acute care and generic skills. This book purposefully maps the Foundation Programme Curriculum in generic skills and includes everything a doctor needs to know about:
- Clinical and communication skills
- Legal and ethical issues
- Clinical governance and patient safety
- Teaching and learning.

To be able to practice medicine effectively, you not only need to know about diseases and treatments, but also vital knowledge that underpins the practice of medicine, whether it be how to structure a consultation, issues about consent, teamwork, evidence-based medicine or how to give effective feedback.

A lot of this knowledge would normally be acquired by observation and 'osmosis'. This takes time and can be inaccurate. Many junior doctors base their knowledge of generic skills on one person's practice or even rumour. Now there is a readily available point of reference.

How to use this book

Essential Guide to Generic Skills is not meant to be read from Chapter 1 to 30. Try starting with a topic that interests you which you can put into practice before returning to another chapter. You might find some chapters are particularly relevant at particular times, or stimulated by specific incidents.

Essential Guide to Generic Skills has been written with the following people in mind:
- Doctors in training
- Medical students
- Other healthcare professionals (e.g. nursing staff, professions allied to medicine)
- Educational supervisors and teachers.

As well as individual readers, we anticipate that this book will be used by teachers of generic skills. The key for teachers who use this book is to read the chapters, use the Further resources and References, a range of teaching methods and imagination to create educational and thought-provoking learning episodes, whether they be tutorials, lectures, workshops or opportunistic teaching.

Generic skills are ultimately learned in the workplace. The key for individual readers is to allow the material to inform and improve their clinical practice.

We have enjoyed learning through writing this book; we hope you enjoy learning through using it!

Nicola Cooper, Kirsty Forrest and Paul Cramp

Acknowledgements

The authors would like to thank their 'other halves', Robert Cooper, Derek Charleston and Gill Cramp, for their support in the writing of this book.

The authors would also like to thank Hayley Oakes for doing the illustrations – we only gave her phrases to work with and she has captured the subjects brilliantly.

Thanks also to our colleagues and friends who have contributed to this book and to all the medical students, nursing staff and junior doctors whose understanding and questions have shaped our writing.

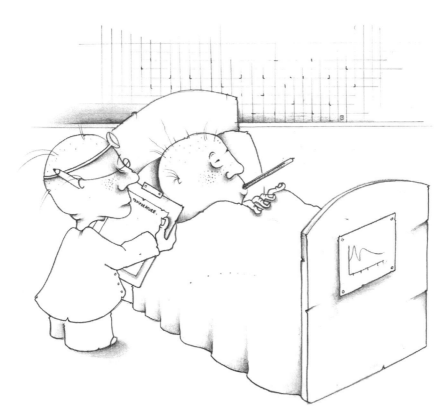

Act.

Disclaimer

Readers are advised that points of law, ethics and professional guidelines change from time to time. The authors and the publishers do not accept responsibility or legal liability for any errors in the text or for the misuse or misapplication of material in this book.

PART I

Clinical and Communication Skills

CHAPTER 1

Professionalism

> **By the end of this chapter you will be able to:**
> - Understand the concept of professionalism
> - Monitor your own professional behaviour
> - Act appropriately if a colleague demonstrates poor professional behaviour
> - Recognise the importance of looking after your own health

Defining professionalism

At the time of writing, professionalism is a highly topical subject. Professionalism is something we can all recognise, yet have difficulty in defining. The General Medical Council's (GMC) 'Good Medical Practice' states that: 'All patients are entitled to good standards of practice and care from their doctors. Essential elements of this are professional competence, good relationships with patients and colleagues, and observance of professional and ethical obligations' [1].

There is an international consensus on the importance of medical professionalism [2]. Unsatisfactory performance in practice is more likely to be due to problems with professional behaviour than lack of knowledge or skills [3]. The importance of professionalism has been reinforced by the recognition that professionalism can and should be taught at medical school [4]. Attitudinal objectives are given equal importance to knowledge and skills during undergraduate studies and increasingly medical schools are including personal and professional development (PPD) programmes in their curricula [5,6].

The Association of American Medical Colleges reached a consensus in 1998 on the broad attributes a doctor needs in order to meet society's expectations of them in the practice of medicine [7]:
- Physicians must be altruistic
- Physicians must be knowledgeable
- Physicians must be skilful
- Physicians must be dutiful.

In other words, being a good doctor is not just about knowledge. The best doctors also demonstrate professionalism and 'Good Medical Practice'. Box 1.1 outlines the GMC's introduction to 'Good Medical Practice' – the UK version of the attributes of a good doctor.

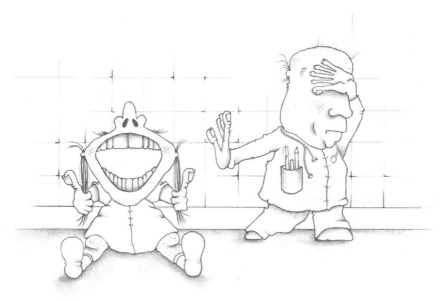

Professionalism.

Box 1.1 Duties of a doctor

Patients must be able to trust doctors with their lives and well-being.
To justify that trust, we as a profession have a duty to maintain a good
standard of practice and care, and to show respect for human life.
In particular, as a doctor you must:
- Make the care of your patient your first concern
- Treat every patient politely and considerately
- Respect patients' dignity and privacy
- Listen to patients and respect their views
- Give patients information in a way they can understand
- Respect the rights of patients to be fully involved in decisions about
  their care
- Keep your professional knowledge and skills up to date
- Recognise the limits of your professional competence
- Be honest and trustworthy
- Respect and protect confidential information
- Make sure that your personal beliefs do not prejudice your
  patients' care
- Act quickly to protect patients from risk if you have good reason to
  believe that you or a colleague may not be fit to practice
- Avoid abusing your position as a doctor
- Work with colleagues in the ways that best serve patients' interests.

> **Box 1.2** A definition of professionalism
>
> Medicine is a vocation in which a doctor's knowledge, clinical skills and judgement are put in service of protecting and restoring human well-being. This purpose is realised through a partnership between patient and doctor, one based on mutual respect, individual responsibility and appropriate accountability.
>
> In their day-to-day practice, doctors are committed to:
> - Integrity
> - Compassion
> - Altruism
> - Continuous improvement
> - Excellence
> - Working in partnership with members of the wider healthcare team.
>
> These values, which underpin the science and practice of medicine, form the basis of a moral contract between the medical profession and society.

The Royal College of Physicians produced a report in 2005, 'Doctors in Society [8]' which examined the concept of medical professionalism. The report defines medical professionalism as a set of values, behaviours and relationships, outlined in Box 1.2.

Professional behaviour

Professional behaviour should be evident in all aspects of a doctor's work and includes team working, ethics, communication skills and the complexity of relationships doctors have with their patients. Professional behaviour and probity are core competencies of the Foundation Curriculum [9] and are listed in Box 1.3.

Practising ethical medicine is a fundamental part of professional behaviour and is discussed in other chapters. It is the integration of good knowledge, skills *and* attitudes in practice that make for a good doctor. All three improve with experience and reflective practice (the ability to pause and think about incidents and learn from them).

One feature of a professional is a high degree of autonomy. As eventual independent practitioners, doctors have to monitor their own professionalism and their own learning. An effective way to do this is through reflective practice, which can turn one's experiences (good and bad) into opportunities for learning. The next time you come across a similar situation, whether clinical, interpersonal or ethical, you will be better prepared to deal with it. Although much reflection takes place informally (e.g. among friends), doctors lead busy lives and unless time is carved out to formally reflect, make a note and think

Box 1.3 Foundation curriculum competencies for professionalism

Doctors should consistently behave with a high degree of professionalism. Overall, a trainee should 'demonstrate an appropriate attitude with consistently high standards of preferred behaviour' and be able to:
- Reflect on learning from practice and experience
- Use a professional and appropriate manner in all communication and medical records
- Ensure all discussion/examination is relevant
- Deal with inappropriate behaviour in patients or carers/relatives
- Respect the rights of vulnerable patient groups
- Recognise the needs of patients and carers/relatives as individuals
- Place the needs of patients above own convenience (without compromising the safety of self or others)
- Be aware of patients' expectations around personal presentation of individual doctors
- Behave with honesty and probity*.

*Probity means 'uprightness' from the Latin word for 'good'.

Box 1.4 Using a portfolio for deliberate reflective practice

New doctors should use their portfolio for more than a record of clinical activity. Use it to record critical incidents and significant events. It is therapeutic and helps untangle the thoughts and actions that took place during an incident and helps determine what more you need to know. Use the following steps:
- Describe the event or incident
- Record how the event or incident challenged your current knowledge, beliefs or understanding
- What have you learned or gained as a result of the event or incident?
- What further learning are you planning to engage with as a result of this event or incident? What resources do you need?
- How will you use this new knowledge or skills in the future?

The ability to reflect consciously upon one's professional practice is important in the development of expertise.

---

about the future, the momentum is lost. 'Deliberate reflective practice' is assisted by a portfolio, which many doctors are now required to keep. Box 1.4 shows how such a portfolio can be used for reflective practice.

It is important that healthcare professionals can recognise poor behaviour and illness in their colleagues. Even good doctors can develop problems, and

Box 1.5 Procedure for acting if a colleague is not fit to practise

If you have grounds to believe that a doctor or other healthcare professional may be putting patients at risk, you must give an honest explanation of your concerns to an appropriate person from the employing authority … following any procedures set by the employer. If there are no appropriate local systems, or local systems cannot resolve the problem, and you remain concerned about the safety of patients, you should inform the relevant regulatory body. If you are not sure what to do, discuss your concerns with an impartial colleague or contact your defence body, a professional organisation or the GMC for advice.

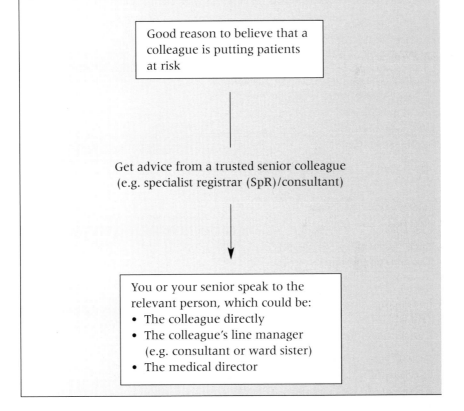

when they do, colleagues seem unequipped to do anything about it. Doctors are often not recognised to be dangerous until they have done considerable damage. Burnout, alcoholism and mental illness are all possible factors (discussed further in Chapter 18). However, doctors have a professional responsibility to protect patients and they must be willing to act, even when colleagues are involved. The GMC has laid out guidelines for doctors to follow in these circumstances (see Box 1.5).

Health

Everyone gets ill and doctors are no different. All doctors and their families should be registered with a general practitioner outside the family, who takes responsibility for their healthcare. Although treating minor ailments or emergency care is acceptable, doctors should generally not treat themselves or their family. 'Corridor' consultations should be avoided. This is common sense, as a proper evaluation cannot be made without a full history, proper examination and access to medical records.

Box 1.6 Useful organisations for doctors with health problems

Sick Doctors Trust
Advice for doctors with drug and alcohol problems
www.sick-doctors-trust.co.uk

National Counselling Service for Sick Doctors
1 Park Square West
London NW1 4LJ
Tel.: 020 7306 372
www.ncssd.org.uk

Association of Anaesthetists Sick Doctor Scheme
Tel.: 020 7631 1650

BMA Counselling Service
Tel.: 0645 200 169

BMA Doctors for Doctors Service
Tel.: 020 7383 6739

British International Doctors' Association
For doctors with cultural and linguistic problems
Tel.: 0161 456 7828
E-mail: oda@doctors.org.uk

Doctors' Support Network
For doctors with mental illness
www.dsn.org.uk

The Doctors' Supportline
Tel.: 0870 765 0001
www.doctorssupportline.org

Independent, confidential and anonymous help for doctors affected by burnout, depression, anxiety, mental distress, work difficulties or family worries. The website contains useful links to a number of other organisations that can offer advice and support.

Doctors are exposed to unique health risks which include:
- Infections (e.g. from needlestick injuries)
- Violence and aggression in the workplace
- Long or unsociable working hours
- Dealing with people's anxiety, suffering, death and bereavement
- Excessive and often chaotic workload
- Perpetual organisational change
- Unrealistic expectations from patients and relatives.

Doctors have higher rates of suicide, divorce and alcohol abuse. They are often reluctant to acknowledge illness because of the pressure this puts on colleagues. Only one-third of junior doctors are registered with a general practitioner [10]. However, it is essential that doctors do what they can to stay healthy, maintain their immunisation status and follow guidelines on health and safety, and infection control.

Medicine can be a stressful profession, which is why the Foundation Curriculum states that new doctors should be able to recognise the signs of stress in themselves and others, and develop healthy coping mechanisms or seek help if appropriate. Many doctors tend towards an obsessive–compulsive personality trait. Understanding this tendency, as well as our other strengths and weaknesses can be helpful in dealing with stress. Some people are naturally insightful, but others who are not can learn through feedback and reflection.

Most deaneries and many other organisations offer confidential support to doctors. Some useful contacts are listed in Box 1.6.

Key points: Professionalism

- Professionalism is at the heart of what it means to be a doctor.
- Doctors have to monitor their own professionalism and their own learning.
- Reflective practice is important in the development of expertise.
- Every doctor should be registered with a general practitioner.
- Doctors are exposed to unique health risks and high levels of stress.
- Doctors should be able to recognise poor professional behaviour and illness in themselves or others and do something about it.

Exercises

- Describe the absence of professionalism. Does this affect patient care?
- How would the definitions of medical professionalism described above impact on your work if everyone were to put them into practice?
- Discuss the European Working Time Directive and professionalism.
- Discuss whether it matters what doctors wear to work.
- Describe how stress affects you and your work.

Self-assessment: Case histories

1 A fellow house officer is always late to work. On-call doctors are always called to his ward to perform routine tasks which should have been done during the normal working day. He graduated at the top of his year and has excellent medical knowledge and confidence, which impresses the consultant during ward rounds. However, colleagues complain that he is lazy, unhelpful and arrogant. You work on the same ward together. Could you do something about this?

2 You are about to start your first senior house officer job, which includes being on-call for the coronary care unit. You are comfortable with most medical emergencies, but are unsure of how to manage cardiac arrhythmias. Do you have a professional responsibility to address this?

3 You have finished clerking in a patient and are writing in the notes. You overhear a nurse on the telephone explaining that he cannot find any doctor to come and see a patient who has developed seriously abnormal vital signs. There seems to be a mix-up as to who is meant to be looking after the patient and the nurse is not getting anywhere. What would you do?

4 You have clerked a patient in with abdominal pain at 2 a.m. and requested some blood tests and X-rays. The patient will be seen on the consultant ward round at 8 a.m. Who is responsible for checking the results?

Self-assessment: Discussion

1 Good doctors are both competent *and* trustworthy. Underperforming doctors rarely have difficulty with theoretical medical knowledge; there is nearly always a problem with professional behaviour (particularly the ability to work in teams, communication skills or what has been termed 'emotional intelligence' – see Further resources). Some people simply do not realise how their behaviour comes across to others and need feedback. Someone needs to speak to this doctor, for example one or two fellow house officers or the ward registrar.

2 One feature of a professional is a high degree of autonomy and the need to monitor one's own learning. A trainee would demonstrate professional behaviour by recognising a learning need and then doing something about it. There are several different ways in which this learning can be done (e.g. reading, asking for a tutorial, going on an Advanced Life Support course).

3 It is professionally unacceptable to say, 'Not my patient' if confronted with someone who is seriously ill. The GMC states that you should 'work with colleagues in ways that best serve patients' interests' and the Foundation Curriculum states that a doctor should 'place the needs of patients above own convenience'. This *is* something to do with you, because you have become aware of an emergency nearby and the fact that there is no other doctor available. You should go and assess the patient, then help the nurse to establish who is responsible for ongoing care.

4 If you see a patient and order some tests, it is your responsibility to see the results of these tests, or hand it over to another doctor if you are going off shift. You should never *assume* that someone else will see the results; there may be an abnormal test result that requires urgent action.

References

1. General Medical Council. *Good Medical Practice*. London, 2001. www.gmc-uk.org/standards/good.htm
2. Sox HC. Medical professionalism in the new millennium: a physician's charter. *Annals of Internal Medicine* 2002; **136**: 243–246.
3. Papadakis MA, Loesr H and Healy K. Early detection and evaluation of professionalism deficiencies in medical students: one school's approach. *Academic Medicine* 2001; **76**: 1100–1106.
4. Cruess SR and Cruess RL. Professionalism must be taught. *British Medical Journal* 1997; **315**: 1674–1677.
5. General Medical Council. *Tomorrow's Doctors*. General Medical Council, London, 1993.
6. Howe A. Twelve tips for developing professional attitudes in training. *Medical Teacher* 2003; **25**: 485–487.
7. Association of American Medical Colleges. *Learning Objectives for Medical Student Education – Guidelines for Medical Schools*. AAMC, 1998. www.aamc.org/meded/msop/start.htm
8. Doctors in Society. Medical professionalism in a changing world. Report of a working party of the Royal College of Physicians Dec 2005. *Clinical Medicine* 2005; **5(6) Suppl 1**: S1–S40.
9. Foundation Programme Committee of the Academy of Medical Royal Colleges. *Curriculum for the Foundation Years in Postgraduate Education and Training*. www.mmc.nhs.uk
10. Department of Health. *Supporting Doctors, Protecting Patients: A Consultation Paper on Preventing, Recognising and Dealing with Poor Clinical Performance of Doctors in the NHS in England*. Department of Health, London, 1999.

Further resources

- BMJ Career Focus theme edition 29 March 2003 on dealing with stress. http://careerfocus.bmjjournals.com
- Boon D and Wardrope J. What should doctors wear in the accident and emergency department? Patients' perception. *Journal of Accident and Emergency Medicine* 1994; **11(3)**: 175–177.
- 'Welcome to the Team' is an introduction for junior doctors working in the NHS and contains all kinds of useful information including how to prevent stress and burnout. www.nhsemployers.org/docs/careers_junior_doctors_brochure.pdf
- Goleman D. *Working with Emotional Intelligence*. Bloomsbury, London, 1999.

CHAPTER 2

The consultation

By the end of this chapter you will be able to:

- Know how to structure consultations effectively
- Understand the value of a patient-centred approach to the consultation
- Know when a chaperone is required
- Understand how to approach complex or difficult consultations
- Conduct effective telephone consultations

The consultation is central to the everyday work of a doctor. The average doctor performs 200,000 consultations in a professional lifetime, so it is worth understanding the consultation and getting it right from the beginning.

Structuring a consultation

The medical model of the consultation is most familiar to doctors. It starts by listening to a patient's story, then asking questions about symptoms and signs, conducting an examination and reaching a diagnosis with or without the help of tests. This traditional clinical method is comprehensive and well researched.

However, in everyday practice this standard approach may not be very effective. Many people, especially the elderly and very young, present with a number of problems that constrictive questioning will not effectively prioritise. The order of presenting complaints may be unrelated to their importance and it is easy to assume that the first problem mentioned is the only one that the patient has brought.

A review of current research has identified the key tasks in a consultation as [1]:

- Eliciting the patient's main problems
- Finding out the patient's perception of these
- Discussing the physical, emotional and social impact of the patient's problems on himself and his family.

You must always try to:

- Tailor the information you give to what the patient wants to know
- Check his understanding
- Elicit the patient's reactions to the information given and his or her main concerns.

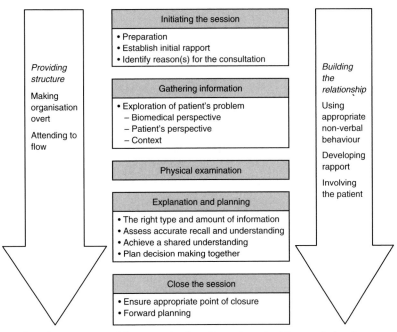

Figure 2.1 Components of the consultation. Reproduced with permission by Radcliffe Publishing. From Ref. [3].

Many different approaches to the medical consultation have been developed over the past 30 years, all trying to enhance the consultation to achieve a better partnership between doctor and patient, which in turn improves health outcomes.

The Cambridge Calgary Guide [2] is one model that applies to most clinical settings and structures the skills which aid doctor–patient communication. It was developed by Kurtz *et al.* [3]. At a basic level this model consists of:

- Initiating the session
- Gathering information
- Physical examination
- Explanation and planning
- Closing the session.

This provides structure, but the focus is much more on building a relationship with the patient as the consultation progresses. These basic blocks can be divided further in to individual skills required in the consultation, as illustrated in Fig. 2.1. Building a relationship is easier if the environment is laid out in a way that facilitates communication, as illustrated in Fig. 2.2.

Initiating the session

Establish a good rapport by introducing yourself and clarifying your role. Make good eye contact, be polite and courteous and allow the patient to speak. Most

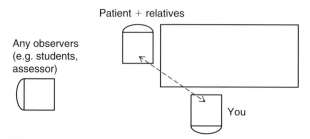

Figure 2.2 Ideal layout of the consultation room. Create a rapport by removing the desk as a barrier. Ensure any observers are on the outside, but able to see and be seen.

Box 2.1 Summarising

Summarising is an useful skill to learn and use appropriately.

Good for patients
- Tells the patient you have been listening
- And that you are interested
- Lets the patient know you understand
- Allows him to go on to his concerns.

Good for doctors
- Maximises the information you gather
- Puts your thoughts in order
- Allows you to change direction if the patient is going off on a tangent
- Allows you to separate disease from illness.

---

patients will decide in the first 90 seconds whether they like you, and by implication, trust you.

Look smart. Research shows that patients feel more comfortable when doctors dress smartly and this correlates with higher patient trust and confidence [4].

Find out the reasons for consultation with open questions and allow patients time to speak without interrupting. Most people do not talk for longer than a minute, so even if you are in a rush this should allow the patient time to cover the issues.

Gathering information

This is the main part of the interview with a lot of information to discover. Explore problems by encouraging the patient to tell the story in his own words. Listen intently and clarify statements which are vague. Summarise what the patient has said as you go along; this will show the patient you have been listening (see Box 2.1).

Basic history taking skills are vital. Good history takers tease out relevant information and ask the right questions. The use of ICE questions (ideas, concerns and expectations) will focus on the patient's perspective and help you understand how his problems are affecting him socially and psychologically:

- Have you any *ideas* about what might be happening?
- What *concerns* you about this problem?
- What are your *expectations* about what we might be able to do for this?

The effort of gathering information about the patient as a whole should start to build a relationship. Picking up on cues, both verbal and non-verbal, will help to develop a rapport, something which is important to many patients.

Explanation and planning

In general, doctors are perceived as poor at giving information to patients. It is important to find out what the patient would like to know and prioritise his information needs, especially when time is short. Giving information in chunks or categories such as the nature of illness, possible causes and treatment options allows people to assimilate it slowly. Summarise what you have said and check for understanding as you go along by asking patients to repeat in their own words what they understand – this helps them remember information.

It is often helpful to provide written information or recommend appropriate websites, so the patient can go over what has been said in his own time.

Planning what happens next requires shared decision making. Try to encourage patients to contribute their own ideas because a shared treatment plan is more likely to be followed.

Closing the session

Again, summarise the whole consultation briefly and clarify what you both have decided to do. Finally, check that the patient is satisfied with the plan and ask if there are any questions or other matters the patient wants to discuss.

The patient-centred approach

The patient-centred approach promotes a partnership between the patient and the doctor. There is a large body of evidence which supports the effectiveness of the patient-centred approach in improving health outcomes for patients. There are a number of models for using this approach, but they all include:

- Concern for the whole person, not just the disease
- Understanding the patient's perspective
- Sharing information, decisions and responsibility between the health professional and the patient.

A simple way of encouraging this type of approach is to think in terms of the agenda of the patient and doctor in the consultation. Sometimes, the agenda of the patient may be completely different from the doctor's (see Fig. 2.3). If the consultation is to be successful, a balance between the two is required [5].

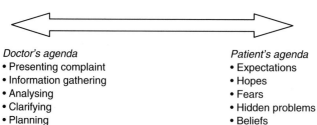

Doctor's agenda
• Presenting complaint
• Information gathering
• Analysing
• Clarifying
• Planning
• Closing the session

Patient's agenda
• Expectations
• Hopes
• Fears
• Hidden problems
• Beliefs

Figure 2.3 Different agendas.

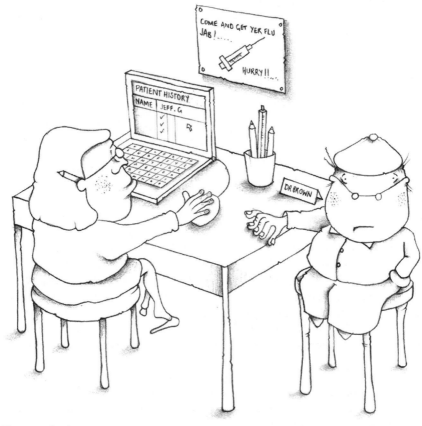

The consultation.

Research shows that if doctors address the patient's agenda as well it can reduce the number of repeat consultations, increase adherence to treatment and reduce the number of complaints [6].

Chaperones

Chaperones are primarily to reassure a patient during what may be an embarrassing or uncomfortable experience. The presence of a chaperone also protects the doctor from allegations of impropriety. Any examination of a patient should include:

- A clear explanation of the purpose and nature of the examination
- The opportunity for the patient to ask questions
- The offer of a chaperone for intimate examinations
- A professional and considerate manner
- Adequate privacy for the patient.

The General Medical Council (GMC) has issued guidelines on the use of chaperones for intimate examinations and states that this should be offered as a matter of routine [7]. Always record the presence of a chaperone and whether the patient declined the offer of a chaperone.

The three-way consultation

Three-way consultations involve a third party such as parent, spouse, interpreter or carer. This can dramatically change the dynamics of a consultation.

In a three-way consultation with a competent patient, you need to bear in mind the following points:

- Focus on the patient and his agenda, not that of the third party
- Develop a good rapport with the patient
- Involve the patient throughout the consultation
- Share decision making by encouraging the patient's own thoughts.

The use of interpreters poses potential problems with confidentiality and consent, and interpreters may not be available at certain times. In reality, relatives often act as interpreters, but relatives can often convey their own opinions rather than acting as a neutral translator. Avoid using friends and relatives as interpreters if possible. If no other interpreter is available, you should emphasise to the relative that you simply want him to translate precisely everything that is said. Always seek the patient's consent before using an interpreter, whoever it may be. Ensure that the interpreter understands the confidential nature of the consultation.

Here are some simple rules to follow when using an interpreter:

- Find out the language the patient speaks (not the nationality).
- Be sensitive to cultural differences – for example, a Muslim lady may not appreciate a male interpreter.
- Introduce the interpreter and emphasise confidentiality.
- Arrange seating in a triangle to allow you to look at the patient directly, so the interpreter is perceived as neutral.
- Talk to the patient, not the interpreter.
- Respond to laughter and non-verbal clues from the patient to help build rapport.

- Try to keep in control of the consultation. This can be tricky especially if the translator and patient know each other. Try not to let the interpreter intervene other than to clarify or check meaning.
- Make use of leaflets and written material. Most National Health Service (NHS) Trusts have excellent material available in local languages explaining procedures and treatments.

Difficult consultations

Patients are a diverse set of people. Some can be rude, hostile and demanding of you and your time, but often this is because they are unwell, anxious, have had bad experiences with doctors before or are simply fed up with the system. Although individual patients and doctors are all different there are useful strategies you can use when faced with a difficult consultation.

As simple as it sounds, first try to be aware of the fact that a patient is making you feel uncomfortable, angry or frustrated. Being aware of such feelings and accepting them can enable you to avoid reacting without thinking. Angry patients may make you feel like getting angry too, but in most cases this is simply counterproductive. Anger on the part of the patient often arises out of frustration – so acknowledge it, apologise for any specific incident and move on. A logical argument or trying to be clever with an angry patient usually makes things worse. If you feel an angry patient is being threatening, abusive or may become violent, call for help. The NHS has a 'zero tolerance' policy on such behaviour.

Sometimes patients are rude rather than angry. Try not to take it personally – either the patient is rude to everyone or they are particularly stressed or anxious. Be professional and do your best to stay polite. When a genuine conflict is arising between you and a patient it can be helpful to pause and acknowledge this explicitly. Identifying there is a difficulty means you are prioritising what matters to the patient and trying to deal with it. Patients often feel worse if they feel you are not listening and do not try to engage emotionally with them.

Discussing a difficult patient with a professional colleague or close friend after the event can help, bearing in mind confidentiality. This is called 'house keeping' – a term coined by Roger Neighbour [8]. Doctors need looking after as well as patients and consultations do not always end when the patient leaves the room. If the consultation went badly, doctors (especially reflective ones) can be left with feelings that need venting or addressing. This helps you to deal with your next patient professionally and efficiently.

Breaking bad news is a particular kind of difficult consultation and is outlined in Box 2.2.

Telephone consultations

In telephone consultations there are no non-verbal cues that help you to judge what the patient is thinking or develop rapport in the same way. It is said that

Box 2.2 Breaking bad news

It is good practice to ask all patients undergoing tests for serious illnesses how they would like to be informed of the results. Some patients prefer to be given bad news alone, but many prefer a close relative to be present. When breaking bad news, make sure you are fully informed of all the facts of the case beforehand, ensure privacy and no interruptions. Breaking bad news occurs in different contexts – you may never have met this person before and are informing them of the sudden cardiac death of a spouse, or you may be talking to a patient and relative you know well, who are already aware that some bad news may be on the way.

A useful framework when breaking bad news is the 10-step approach [9]:

1 Preparation – know the facts and who will be present; ensure privacy and no interruptions; sit down together
2 Explore what is already known
3 'Test the waters' to see if more information is wanted
4 Some patients cope by denial, which is rarely permanent; allow this
5 Before the bad news, fire a warning shot, for example, 'as you know you have been having tests for a shadow on your lung, because we were worried it could be something serious'
6 When you give bad news, use clear and simple language; say the word 'cancer' if that is what you mean and avoid euphemisms
7 Elicit concerns and allow time for questions
8 Allow ventilation of feelings, but never say you understand how someone feels
9 Summarise and plan
10 Further talks are often needed, so offer yourself or someone else available for this.

When breaking bad news, go slowly and be comfortable with silence. Try to tailor the information to the patient's needs and gauge how and what information the patient wants to know. Try to understand the patient's perspective and make decisions together.

Nearly all NHS Trusts run courses in breaking bad news. Make the most of opportunities to watch senior colleagues break bad news and learn from this.

only 30% of your range of communication skills can be used over the telephone, so communication skills have to be more explicit.

The particular skills required for a successful telephone consultation are active listening, systematic history taking and summarising. Take the call in a quiet room where you can hear clearly and will not be disturbed. Have the patient's notes to hand and a pen and paper. Check the other person's identity and give a 'verbal handshake' by introducing yourself and sounding friendly.

Telephone consultations are structured in a similar way to face-to-face consultations, but you must ensure that you are in a position to give advice before you do so. In many cases it is necessary to see and examine a patient before being able to offer proper advice, and if that is the case, you should say so.

Finally, consultations require a high quality of information exchange between you, your patients and their families and it can be frustrating and upsetting if consultations do not go according to plan. It is guaranteed that not all of them will. Often time is short and you must prioritise, leaving some of the patient's questions for another time. Some patients may have unrealistic expectations or you may be having a bad day.

By making time to reflect on your consultations and your response to the ones that do not go well, you will become more equipped to cope with the everyday stresses of being a doctor. Nobody is perfect.

Key points: The consultation

- The Cambridge Calgary Guide is a useful structure which also fosters building relationships with patients.
- Summarising is an useful skill to learn and use appropriately.
- ICE questions can be used to find out the patient's perspective.
- Shared decision making is more likely to be effective.
- Be aware that patients often have a different agenda to the doctor.
- In three-way consultations with a competent patient, focus on the patient.
- Difficult consultations can be stressful – talk things over with a colleague.

Exercises

- Try structuring your consultations deliberately in the way described above. Does this make a difference?
- Self appraisal is a skill all doctors have to learn. Try seeing one of your consultations through the eyes of the patient. How would you rate yourself?
- Ask a knowledgeable colleague to sit in on some of your consultations and ask for feedback. Videoing consultations for this purpose (with the patient's consent) is commonplace in general practice.

References

1. Maguire P and Piceathly C. Key communication skills and how to acquire them. Clinical review. *British Medical Journal* 2002; **325**: 697–700.
2. Kurtz SM and Silverman JD. Cambridge Calgary Guide: A guide to the medical interview. *Education* 1996; **30**: 83–89.
3. Kurtz SM, Silverman JD and Draper J. *Teaching and Learning Communication Skills in Medicine*, 2nd edn. Radcliffe Publishing, Oxford, 2005.

4. Nair BR, Attia BR, Mears SR and Hitchcock KI. Evidence-based physicians' dressing: a crossover trial. *Medical Journal of Australia* 2002; **177**: 681–682.
5. Tate P. *The Doctor's Communication Handbook*, 4th edn. Radcliffe Publishing, Oxford, 2003.
6. Abdel-Tawab N and Roter DL. The relevance of client-centred communication to family planning settings in developing countries: lessons from the Egyptian experience. *Social Science and Medicine* 2002; **54**: 1347–1368.
7. General Medical Council. *Intimate Examinations*. www.gmc.org.uk
8. Neighbour R. *The Inner Consultation*, 2nd edn. Radcliffe Publishing, Oxford, 2005.
9. Kaye P. *Breaking Bad News: A 10 Step Approach*. EPL Publishing, Northampton, 1995.

Further resource

- Kurtz SM, Silverman JD and Draper J. *Skills for Communicating with Patients*, 2nd edn. Radcliffe Publishing, Oxford, 2005.

CHAPTER 3
Health promotion

By the end of this chapter you will be able to:

- Use a number of resources to help patients
- Know the effect of environment and lifestyle as risk factors for disease
- Understand the impact of obesity
- Understand the issues around smoking cessation
- Understand the effects of alcohol on health
- Know about screening

When doctors give clear information and involve patients in a mutually acceptable management plan, that plan is more likely to be followed and in turn leads to better health outcomes. There is a wealth of patient societies, websites, specialist nurses and educational leaflets that doctors can and should use to help in this process. An example is shown in Box 3.1.

Box 3.1 Case history

A 20-year-old student is diagnosed with juvenile myoclonic epilepsy, a common form of idiopathic generalised epilepsy. Lifestyle factors are very important in this condition, as seizures are commonly precipitated by lack of sleep, stress and alcohol. The patient continues to have seizures due to lifestyle triggers, despite taking medication. What resources are available to you, his doctor, to help educate the patient about his condition?

- Information leaflets
- Epilepsy action: www.epilepsy.org.uk
- A specialist colleague
- Your Trust's epilepsy nurse specialist whom the patient can contact
- The patient's family.

The environment and lifestyle as risk factors for disease

Disease occurs as a result of interactions between a harmful agent, the environment and people. As modern medicine allows people to live longer and longer with their diseases, prevention of disease is becoming more important from an economic as well as a humanitarian point of view. Prevention strategies can be targeted at the agent, the environment or people themselves. For example, a vaccine has been developed against the causative agent of cervical cancer, the human papilloma virus. But action targeting the social environment and individuals is also required for prevention, since this is a sexually transmitted disease.

Preventative action is sometimes classified as primary, secondary or tertiary. Primary prevention is preventing the disease from occurring in the first place. This includes immunisation and health promotion. The improvements in health in the western world over the past 200 years are mainly due to improvements in sanitation and social conditions rather than specific medical interventions [1]. However, there are modern day examples of drugs used in primary prevention, for example the use of statins in high-risk groups.

Secondary prevention includes measures to prevent further progression of disease once it has been detected. A well-known example of secondary prevention is the use of aspirin in angina or after a transient ischaemic attack.

Tertiary prevention is disease limitation by modifying risk factors and instituting rehabilitation.

The Department of Health published a public health white paper in 2004 entitled 'Choosing health: making healthier choices easier'. The introduction to the white paper makes the points that:
- A woman born in 1900 could expect to live to the age of 50 years. Today it is 80 years
- The UK faces new health challenges: the effects of obesity, smoking and alcohol are among them
- Ill health is linked to poverty.

The white paper identifies seven key areas for public health action:
1 Obesity
2 Smoking
3 Alcohol
4 Sexual health (sexually transmitted disease are on the increase)
5 Mental health (one in four general practitioners' (GPs) consultations are related to mental health and dementia is increasing with an increasing elderly population)
6 Accidents, including falls in the elderly (a major cause of morbidity and death)
7 Substance misuse (around 1 million people use class A drugs in the UK).

In today's consumer society, public health strategies have to take into account people's desire for information, individualism and partnership – quite a challenge. At government level, improving school dinners, encouraging sport,

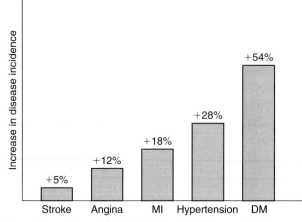

Figure 3.1 The estimated impact of obesity by 2023 (from 1998). MI: myocardial infarction; DM: type 2 diabetes mellitus. Reproduced with permission from the Department of Health.

providing cycle lanes and smoking legislation are a few examples of public health measures. For healthcare professionals, it is a matter of being aware of our duty to promote health as well as treat disease and to recognise opportunities to promote health.

Obesity

Figure 3.1 shows the estimated impact by 2023 of increasing obesity in the population. Currently, it is estimated that at least one-third of adults will be obese by 2020. The costs to the UK economy in treating the consequences of obesity, sickness absence and premature death is £3.7 billion per year.

Obesity is more common in people of Asian origin, Black people and lower social groups. Improved leisure facilities, physical education in schools, limits on food advertising to children, improved food labelling and better education for healthcare staff are proposed public health measures. Physically active people have a 30% reduced risk of premature death and a 50% reduced risk of major chronic diseases such as heart disease, stroke, diabetes and cancer. Yet six out of ten men and seven out of ten women in the UK are not active enough to benefit their health. One in three deaths from cancer and coronary heart disease are due to a poor diet. Consuming at least five portions of fruit and vegetables per day can reduce the risk of heart disease, stroke and cancer by up to 20%. Reducing the average salt intake of the population to 6 g/day would reduce hypertension and strokes in the population by 15%.

Losing 10 kg of weight reduces total mortality by 20% as well as helping people feel better. Low-calorie, or low-fat diets, increased physical activity or a combination of diet and exercise are effective in reducing weight. Education for health professionals in primary care is also effective [2]. The National

---

Box 3.2 The FRAMES model for brief interventions

This chapter discusses brief interventions for three common public health problems: obesity, smoking and alcohol. Brief interventions have the following characteristics:
- *Feedback*: of your assessment to the patient
- *Responsibility*: advise the patient that the problem is his responsibility
- *Advice*: clear, written or verbal
- *Menu*: offer a range of options which can help
- *Empathy*: be warm and understanding
- *Self-efficacy*: encourage the patient's self-efficacy for change (optimism).

Institute for Clinical Excellence is scheduled to publish guidance on the prevention, identification and management of obesity in 2007.

Doctors have a duty to inform patients of the significant health risks of obesity and give them information and further resources which can help them do something about it. Brief interventions are outlined in Box 3.2.

Smoking

Currently around 10 million adults in England smoke (one quarter of all adults). Nearly 10% of 11–15 year olds smoke. Smoking is the UK's greatest cause of preventable illness. More than 120,000 people die from smoking each year. Yet 70% of smokers say they want to give up. Banning smoking in enclosed public places, limiting tobacco advertising, advertising campaigns and smoking cessation services are all current public health measures to reduce smoking in the UK.

Evidence from meta-analyses shows that brief interventions by doctors in the course of routine care increase the chances of a smoker quitting, and follow-up appointments or support from another healthcare provider has a small additional benefit. The use of nicotine replacement therapy increases the chance of stopping smoking by 80%. Most of this evidence comes from primary care, and there is no evidence to suggest that doctors, nurses or psychologists are better than each other. Interestingly, there is no evidence that brief interventions for hospital in-patients work, unless support extends beyond discharge [3].

A brief intervention literally means a conversation about smoking. However, one study looked at patient's perceptions of doctor's attempts to discuss smoking. It found that if doctors are to raise the subject of smoking, patients preferred a respectful tone, sensitivity to whether the person was ready to give up smoking or not, understanding the patient as an individual and a supportive attitude [4]. The majority of smokers anticipated that they would receive advice about smoking when attending for healthcare and pointed out that the negative effects of smoking are already well known to smokers. The authors concluded that, rather than ritualistic interventions, doctors should seek to understand what the patient thinks about his smoking first and then tailor their approach to the type of patient.

Alcohol

Around 6 million people in the UK regularly consume more alcohol than the recommended limits and this includes young people and the elderly. Alcohol is strongly linked to domestic violence, violent crime, days off work and one-third of attendances at Accident and Emergency departments [5]. Approximately 20% of patients admitted to hospital for illnesses unrelated to alcohol drink to excess [6]. In one study, 6.2% of all admissions to one hospital over a 2-month period were directly attributable to alcohol, and 3000 extra new outpatient visits in the subsequent 18 months [7]. The incidence is much higher for head injuries.

One unit is 8 g of alcohol which is equivalent to half a pint of ordinary beer or cider, one quarter of a pint of extra strong beer or cider, a small (100 ml) glass of wine or a single pub measure (25 ml) of spirits.

The recommended limit for alcohol is 21 units/week for men and 14 units/week for women. A heavy drinker is a man who drinks more than 50 units/week or a woman who drinks more than 35 units/week. A binge drinker is a man who regularly drinks more than 10 units/session or a woman who drinks more than 7 units/session.

It is important to understand that many people drink alcohol to excess but cannot be described as 'alcoholics' – people who have a compulsion to drink, who are dependent on alcohol and suffer withdrawal symptoms.

Brief interventions in a general practice setting have been shown to reduce alcohol consumption, especially in men [8]. Unlike smoking, alcohol in moderation has been shown to have beneficial effects, and this makes public health measures at reducing alcohol consumption more complex.

Asking about alcohol intake is an important part of history taking, yet one study found that only one-third of clerk-ins contained an adequate alcohol history [9]. The CAGE questions are taught in medical school, but only detect severe alcohol intake or alcohol dependence (Box 3.3).

Currently, despite the fact that patients with alcohol problems are common in hospital, healthcare staff tend to ignore it and focus on the presenting complaint instead. If alcohol problems manifest during the hospital stay, for example delirium tremens, this is managed by junior medical staff inadequately [6].

Best practice around the UK includes identifying problem drinkers, offering brief interventions, having an alcohol service including a specialist nurse, implementing staff training and protocols for how to deal with acute alcohol problems, for example withdrawal, and onward referral to appropriate services.

Screening

The UK National Screening Committee [10] advises the government on screening programmes in the UK. Conditions are suitable for a screening programme

---

Box 3.3 The CAGE questions

- Have you ever felt you should *cut* down on your drinking?
- Have people ever *annoyed* you by commenting on your drinking?
- Have you ever felt *guilty* about your drinking?
- Have you ever had a drink first thing in the morning (*eye opener*) to steady your nerves or get rid of a hangover?

---

if they meet internationally recognised criteria, originally developed by the World Health Organisation. These are:
- The condition is an important health problem
- Its natural history is well understood
- It is detectable at an early stage
- Treatment at an early stage improves outcome
- A simple, safe and validated test exists
- The test is acceptable to the population being screened
- Adequate facilities exist to cope with any abnormalities detected
- Screening is done at repeated intervals when the onset is insidious
- The chance of harm is less than the chance of benefit
- Screening is cost effective.

Screening is a public health service in which a targeted population is offered an intervention or test to identify those who may benefit from further tests or treatment. Screening is different to normal healthcare practice in that apparently healthy people are targeted. Screening is not infallible and does not guarantee protection against a disease. All tests have a false positive and a false negative rate and it is important that patients understand the limitations of screening programmes.

Currently in the UK the following conditions are screened for:
- Breast cancer in women aged 50–64 years every 3 years and women aged 65 years and over by request.
- Cervical cancer in women aged 20–64 years every 5 years.
- All neonates are screened for phenylketonuria and have a physical examination.

Key points: Health promotion

- People are now living longer with their diseases, making health promotion an important priority for the National Health Service (NHS).
- The epidemics of obesity, smoking and alcohol abuse are three major examples where health promotion is vital.
- Brief interventions by doctors do make a difference.
- Offering help and further resources help even more.
- Patients are more receptive to a non-judgemental attitude during brief interventions.
- Screening can benefit a population if the condition and test meet certain criteria.

- Newly registered patients and those not seen within 3 years in GP practices are screened for cardiovascular risk factors.
- Every patient over the age of 75 years in GP practices receives a general health screen every 12 months.
- All women receiving antenatal care are offered a HIV test.

Other conditions which are being evaluated for screening in the future include colorectal cancer, abdominal aortic aneurysm and chlamydia infection.

Exercises

- How often do you provide further resources to your patients, for example leaflets, websites and specialist nurse services?
- Find out what services there are in your NHS Trust for smokers who would like help to give up.
- Role play a brief intervention with an obese person, smoker or heavy drinker.
- Doctors have a high alcohol intake compared to the rest of the population. How much alcohol do you drink per week?
- Talk about your experiences with alcohol problems in patients. What do you think your department could do to change this?

References

1. McKeown T. *The Role of Medicine: Mirage, Dream or Nemesis?* Princeton University Press, Princeton, NJ, 1992.
2. The management of obesity and overweight. An analysis of reviews of diet, physical activity and behavioural approaches. www.publichealth.nice.org.uk
3. Smoking interventions – review 25 Jan 2006. www.publichealth.nice.org.uk
4. Butler C, Pill R and Stott NCH. Qualitative study of patients' perceptions of doctors' advice to quite smoking. Implications for opportunistic health promotion. *British Medical Journal* 1998; **316**: 1878–1881.
5. Holt S, Stewart IC, Dixon JMJ, Elton RA *et al.* Alcohol and the emergency service patient. *British Medical Journal* 1980; **281**: 638–640.
6. Report of a working party of the Royal College of Physicians. *Alcohol – Can the NHS Afford It? Recommendations for a Coherent Alcohol Strategy for Hospitals*. Royal College of Physicians, London, 2001.
7. Pirmohamed M, Brown C, Owens L, Luke C *et al.* The burden of alcohol misuse on an inner-city general hospital. *Quarterly Journal of Medicine* 2000; **93**: 291–295.
8. Freemantle N, Gill P, Godfrey C, Long A *et al.* Brief interventions and alcohol use. *Quality in Health Care* 1993; **2**: 267–273.
9. Barrison IG, Viola L and Murray-Lyon IM. Do housemen take an adequate drinking history? *British Medical Journal* 1980; **281**: 1040.
10. UK National Screening Committee. www.nsc.nhs.uk

CHAPTER 4

Clinical reasoning

> **By the end of this chapter you will be able to:**
> - Know the processes involved in clinical reasoning
> - Understand how to interpret diagnostic tests
> - Know how novices and experts differ in reasoning strategies
> - Be aware of biases in clinical reasoning

Modernising Medical Careers [1] and the European Working Time Directive have had the effect of introducing more structured, shorter postgraduate medical training in the UK. This has rekindled an interest in clinical reasoning, since experts think in a very different way to novices, and there is a great deal of interest in understanding how we can teach effective reasoning skills, rather than this being something that is simply absorbed (or not) with time.

There are two broad models of clinical reasoning:
1 Analytical, whereby pieces of information (symptoms, signs and test results) are linked to one or more diagnoses. Hypotheses are formed and then tested.
2 Pattern recognition, whereby the current case is compared to previous ones, sometimes subconsciously.

The ability to use pattern recognition increases with clinical experience. However, these two models of clinical reasoning can occur simultaneously and there is some evidence to suggest that teaching both models to trainees can increase their diagnostic accuracy [2].

Analytical reasoning

The analytical model of clinical reasoning is familiar to doctors. When a patient presents with chest pain, there is a list of possible causes which have been learned. As further information is gathered one diagnosis becomes more likely and others less likely. This is not as easy as it sounds. A careful history, accurate physical examination, the ability to interpret clinical findings and the correct use and interpretation of tests is required.

Even with 21st century technology, *the history and examination form the major part of how doctors make a diagnosis*. Medical students are traditionally taught that history contributes 80%, physical examination 10% and tests another 10% [3]. An up-to-date study found that history and physical examination alone led to

Box 4.1 A case of probabilities

A 40-year-old male is admitted to hospital with vague abdominal pains and a fever. He drinks alcohol to excess. His white cell count is slightly raised and he has proteinuria. A diagnosis of urinary tract infection is made and he is started on antibiotics. What kind of analytical reasoning might follow the presentation of this case?

- Urinary tract infections are uncommon in 40-year-old men
- Proteinuria can be caused by fever and is not diagnostic of urinary tract infection
- Gastritis and pancreatitis are more common causes of vague abdominal pains in males who drink alcohol to excess
- Pancreatitis commonly causes fever
- A serum amylase should be requested

(This patient did have acute pancreatitis).

a correct diagnosis in 70% of cases [4]. Yet when the clinical skills of trainees are assessed, there are often significant omissions in the history or physical examination [5].

In the analytical model, a doctor makes a diagnosis based on probabilities – firstly the clinical probability (based on patient characteristics, history and examination) and then probability adjusted by tests. Knowledge from textbooks, review articles or clinical prediction rules are important but not enough to generate a clinical probability. Experience is also required, because diseases vary far more in their attributes in real life than those described. Using probabilities to help make a diagnosis is referred to as the Bayesian approach after 'Bayes theorem' in mathematics, which deals with probabilities. A Bayesian approach uses all relevant information to estimate the prior probability of a disease before interpreting gathered information [6] (see Box 4.1).

Clinical (pre-test) probability is very important. Without it, a diagnostic test cannot be interpreted. For example, a headache in a 25-year-old is most unlikely to be due to temporal arteritis and a raised erythrocyte sedimentation rate (ESR) is likely to be due to something else, but the diagnosis is much more likely if there are typical symptoms and signs in a 75-year-old lady.

Interpreting diagnostic tests

Having stressed the importance of the history and physical examination, tests also play an important role in the diagnostic process. However, tests can lie! It is important to always look at the patient when interpreting any test, and to understand some key things about diagnostic tests:

- Sensitivity and specificity
- Normal values
- Operating characteristics

Box 4.2 Sensitivity and specificity

- Sensitivity is the ability of a test to pick up true positives, whereas specificity is the ability of a test to rule out true negatives.
- Tests that are very sensitive are good at picking up diseases, whereas tests that are very specific are good at ruling out diseases.
- All tests have a sensitivity and a specificity. Tests do not make a diagnosis; doctors do.

- Factors other than disease which influence test results
- Unexpected test results.

Sensitivity and specificity

The probability of a disease depends on the clinical (pre-test) probability and then the sensitivity and specificity of the test [7]. Sensitivity and specificity is defined in Box 4.2.

Doctors have to make decisions without definitive information a lot of the time because there is no such thing as a perfect diagnostic test. One of the characteristics of a medical professional is 'judgement in the face of uncertainty [8]'. Even with a good test, which has 90% sensitivity and 90% specificity, 10% of patients with the disease will have a normal test result and 10% of patients without the disease will have an abnormal test result.

A good example of pre-test probability, sensitivity and specificity is in the diagnosis of pulmonary embolism (PE) using ventilation–perfusion (V/Q) scanning. The prospective investigation of pulmonary embolism diagnosis (PIOPED) study involved 1000 patients and assessed clinical probability with sensitivity and specificity of V/Q scanning in the diagnosis of PE, compared to the gold standard pulmonary angiography [9].

Before testing, patients were classified into low, intermediate or high clinical probability for PE:
- *Low clinical probability*: no risk factors and another obvious diagnosis which could account for the symptoms and signs.
- *High clinical probability*: risk factors and no other obvious diagnosis which could account for the symptoms and signs.
- *Intermediate probability*: not falling easily in to either of the above categories.
Patients then underwent V/Q scanning and pulmonary angiography and the results are shown in Fig. 4.1.

Patients with a normal V/Q scan were unlikely to have a PE on angiography and patients with a high-probability V/Q scan were likely to have a PE on angiography. But this diagnostic certainty applied only to some patients. As you can see, a patient with a high clinical probability of a PE and a low probability V/Q scan still had a 40% chance of having a PE, a diagnosis which is potentially fatal if untreated.

V/Q scan results (probability)				
		'Non-diagnostic'		
	Normal/very low	Low	Intermediate	High
Clinical probability				
Low	2	4	16	56
Intermediate	6	16	28	88
High	0	40	66	96

Note: Computed tomography pulmonary angiography is widely accepted as the best way to diagnose PE nowadays as pulmonary angiography carries a risk of complications.

Figure 4.1 Percentage of patients with PE (on pulmonary angiography) categorised by their clinical probability and V/Q scan results.

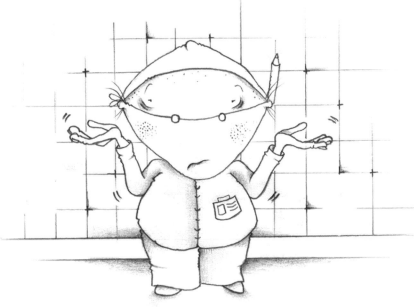

Clinical reasoning.

This example illustrates how the likelihood of a diagnosis changes if the clinical (pre-test) probability changes, even though the test result remains the same. It also gives a useful example of how to classify patients in to low, intermediate or high clinical probability.

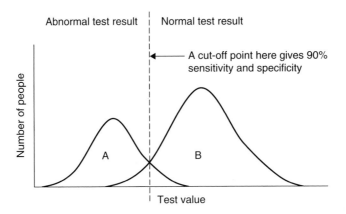

Abnormal test result | Normal test result

A cut-off point here gives 90% sensitivity and specificity

Number of people

A

B

Test value

With any normal distribution, there are people whose test results lie at the extremes, but this does not mean they have a disease.

In this example, moving the cut-off point to the right would increase the chances of picking up abnormals (increase sensitivity) but at the same time increase the rate of false positives (reduce specificity).

Figure 4.2 Interpretation of a 'normal' test result (A: people with the disease; B: people without the disease).

Normal values

It is important to understand that there is an overlap between test results in patients who have and do not have a disease. However, it is necessary to define a cut-off point at which the test is said to be normal or abnormal. This cut-off point is chosen to minimise the number of false positives and false negatives. Fig. 4.2 illustrates this.

To make things more complicated, tests are not necessarily 'positive' or 'negative'. A disease may evolve over time, and a test may become *more* abnormal.

Operating characteristics

Before ordering a test, it is important to be aware of certain operating characteristics of that test. This refers to the method of performing the test. For example, measuring spirometry requires that the patient be able to hear, understand and co-operate with instructions. Exercise electrocardiogram testing is inappropriate in left bundle branch block or in a patient who cannot walk.

Some conditions are paroxysmal. In epilepsy, 50% of patients have a normal electroencephalogram (EEG) between attacks. (Sometimes an abnormality does not mean disease – people without clinical epilepsy have occasional abnormal discharges on the EEG.)

Factors other than disease which influence test results

Clinicians also need to be aware of other things which influence test results, such as:
- Age
- Ethnicity

- Sex
- Pregnancy
- Body position
- Chance
- Spurious (*in vitro*) results
- Laboratory error.

For example, men have slightly different test values to women. Many test results are normal in pregnancy which would be considered abnormal at other times, for example, anaemia, raised alkaline phosphatase. Laboratory error can be the result of technical or human failure, for example uncalibrated analysers or taking blood from the drip arm.

Unexpected test results

When an unexpected test result crops up, pause before acting. Most unexpectedly abnormal test results lie just outside the normal range. If you receive a test result which is grossly abnormal *and* does not fit the clinical picture, it is likely that the test is wrong. Conversely, a normal test result in the face of an obvious clinical abnormality should also make you question the result (see Box 4.3).

Thresholds

Another important consideration in making a diagnosis is whether to do a test at all. If the test will make no difference to the probability of a disease, should the test be done? Tests are most helpful when they will change the management of a patient's illness. Whether to perform a test or start treatment depends on the 'therapeutic threshold'. The threshold concept combines factors such as test characteristics, risks and availability of tests, and the risks and benefits of treatment. The point at which all these factors are evenly weighed is the therapeutic threshold. If a test or treatment for a disease is effective and low risk, one would have a lower threshold for requesting these. But if a test or treatment is less effective or high risk, one requires greater confidence in the clinical diagnosis and potential benefits first.

Box 4.3 An unexpected result

An elderly lady was admitted after a fall. She had hurt her right hip and could not weight bear. On examination the hip was shortened, externally rotated and extremely painful to move. It was a clinical fractured neck of femur. Her pelvic and lateral hip X-rays were normal, so she was admitted to a medical ward. The medical specialist registrar (SpR) who examined her the next day declared there was a fracture and re-ordered the X-rays which this time showed the fracture clearly. By now the patient was on the wrong ward, which led to a delay in taking her to theatre.

Sometimes testing is of no benefit when the disease is clinically apparent but there is no effective treatment option, for example, arranging a biopsy in a patient dying of incurable cancer.

Pattern recognition

Studies of human cognition suggest that problem solving strategies depend on the clinical problem being addressed and the expertise of the clinician. Analytical reasoning can be applied to many clinical settings, but is often inefficient and sometimes less accurate. Experienced doctors quickly home in on a problem by recognising patterns, formulating problems in chunks, gathering relevant data in context and applying familiar solutions. In other words, novices see the trees (and often get distracted by them) and experts see the whole wood. However, when there is no recognisable pattern, experts also use an analytical approach in order to gather information 'from first principles'.

You may have witnessed pattern recognition, when a senior doctor seems to pluck the right diagnosis out of thin air. This intuitive type of reasoning means it is often hard for the expert to describe how he got there. We often hear of people talking about 'gut feeling', but in reality it is based on recognising patterns from a vast databank of previous experiences.

The processes of deliberate practice, building up an experience bank, getting accurate and timely feedback and reflection are the ways in which novices acquire expertise in any area, including clinical reasoning [10].

Bias in clinical reasoning

Doctors often have to make rapid decisions based on gathered information. The best way to gather information is to ask the right questions, interpret the answers correctly and know when to stop searching further [11]. This is not as easy as it sounds – you may have observed the difference between a medical student and an experienced doctor taking a history. There are also pitfalls, or biases, that can easily be made when gathering information. These are [12]:

- Similar does not mean the same. Sometimes doctors can assume that because something is similar to other things in a certain category, it is a member of that category. Studies have found that novices tend to give too much weight to one piece of information or do not take in to account probabilities when making a diagnosis. Just because the answer fits does not mean it is the answer.
- Doctors may emphasise things they are more familiar with, regardless of whether it is factually accurate. For example, if you are an epilepsy expert, then everyone who collapses might have epilepsy.
- Overconfidence is a particular problem with novices. Junior doctors do not know what they do not know. Hasty diagnoses may result, and subsequent suboptimal treatment. It is good practice to be aware of your own limitations and seek the advice of experienced colleagues.

- Doctors may have a tendency to look for and remember information that fits with pre-existing expectations and ignore evidence which contradicts this. For example, when taking a history, one might ask questions designed to confirm an expectation and then stop prematurely, missing important information. The power of suggestion is evident in the UK system of 'multiple clerk-ins'. A patient may be wrongly labelled on admission, and this label is perpetuated because subsequent doctors assume it is correct.
- There may be a tendency to perceive two events as causally related, when there is no evidence that this is the case. For example, patients might get better every time you prescribe peppermint water for pneumonia, leading to the incorrect belief that peppermint water has a therapeutic effect in this condition.

To summarise, clinical reasoning is a skill which takes years to develop and is a vital part of what it means to be a doctor. Diagnosis is not necessarily a one-off event. Information can be gained over a period of time, and diagnostic hypotheses change as new information is gathered. Especially in difficult, or 'grey' cases, diagnosis is often a *process*. In an emergency, or in serious illness, treatment may be required even when the diagnosis is unknown. This can make some doctors uneasy, as well as their patients, who may not be comfortable with the inherent uncertainty in the practice of medicine. This is when communication skills become more important.

Key points: Clinical reasoning

- There are two broad models of clinical reasoning: analytical and pattern recognition
  - The analytical model of clinical reasoning involves probabilities
  - Pattern recognition is commonly used by experts.
- The history and examination form the major part of how doctors make a diagnosis.
- The probability of a disease depends on the clinical (pre-test) probability and the sensitivity and specificity of the test.
- Tests can mislead – doctors need to understand how to use and interpret tests.
- Doctors need to be aware of potential pitfalls, or biases, in their clinical reasoning.

Exercises

- Take one case where you took the history, performed the examination and formulated a management plan and analyse it in terms of the analytical model of clinical reasoning (clinical probability, the characteristics of the tests and treatment thresholds).
- Describe times when you have used or seen pattern recognition at work.

- Talk about scenarios where you have seen pitfalls, or biases, occur in the clinical reasoning process.
- Talk about your experience of and response to uncertainty in the practice of medicine.

Self-assessment: Case histories

Use the following case histories to think about clinical reasoning. Are there aspects of analytical reasoning, pattern recognition, thresholds or biases in these histories?

1 A 16-year-old girl was admitted with three collapses in the same day. The initial clerk-in said 'seizures'. She was observed to briefly lose consciousness and jerk her limbs. Moreover, her mother reports that epilepsy runs in the family. In this context, you are asked to clerk-in the patient on the medical admissions unit. What are your thoughts at this point?

You see the girl with her mother and take a history. The mother describes how the patient had not been feeling well with a urinary tract infection and passed out whilst sitting on the toilet that morning. Mother heard a shout and found her daughter unresponsive on the floor, looking pale and she could not feel a pulse. She dialled 999. The girl came round quickly. In the Accident and Emergency (A&E) department, the girl was observed to flop and briefly lose consciousness whilst having blood taken. She was sent to the waiting area where she vomited. As she vomited she passed out and was observed to go rigid briefly and jerk her limbs. She recovered quickly again. What are your thoughts as to the diagnosis?

It emerges, on further questioning, that the girl is prone to fainting at the sight of blood, needles and vomit. Her father had seizures related to alcohol rather than epilepsy. What is the diagnosis now?

2 A 70-year-old man is admitted after a collapse in church. He was standing for a long time when he felt light-headed. Witnesses said he went pale before passing out briefly. Now he is back to normal. He is on medicines for hypertension. A D-dimer is requested as part of his blood tests. It comes back raised. What is the interpretation of this and what further tests are needed?

3 A 50-year-old lady complains of breathlessness and she is wheezy on examination, especially at night. She has been started on treatment for an exacerbation of chronic obstructive pulmonary disease (nebulisers, steroids and antibiotics) but is not getting better after several days. Apart from a very wheezy chest and a respiratory rate of 24/minute, her other vital signs are normal. Her peak flow is 70% of predicted. What do you do now?

You ask someone more experienced to look at the patient and you go over the history, examination and test results again together. In the medical notes, the history says that the patient never smoked. She has type 2 diabetes, angina and hypertension. Her electrocardiogram shows Q waves in leads V1 and V2. The chest X-ray shows clear lung fields and cardiomegaly.

Your experienced colleague recognises a pattern. What is a more likely diagnosis?

Self-assessment: Discussion

1 A tilt test was performed which was positive and the family was given general advice about vaso-vagal syncope. This is an example of seeing the trees rather than the entire wood, focusing on jerking in the history and assuming the diagnosis of seizures. In addition, a pre-existing label has been assigned to the patient and this can prevent you from exploring other possibilities or cause you to ignore obvious information which goes against that diagnosis. Although the diagnosis of vaso-vagal syncope is clinically obvious after a proper history, this is an example where a simple, safe test was performed in order to provide reassurance to the patient. However, like all tests, the tilt test can be negative in people prone to vaso-vagal syncope and can induce fainting in normal people. However, in the context of the high clinical (pre-test) probability, the positive test confirms the clinical impression. Notice that an expert taking this history would elicit information 'on further questioning' because of pattern recognition.

2 This is an example where you need to understand the nature of the test to be able to interpret the information correctly. The D-dimer is a very specific test but not very sensitive. In other words, it is of value when it is negative and good at excluding diagnoses which are of low clinical probability, but when it is raised it is of no diagnostic value. Many conditions (not necessarily diseases) cause an increase in D-dimer levels. Take the information about D-dimer out of the case history. Would pulmonary embolism even cross your mind?

3 This patient improved dramatically after starting a nitrate at night for heart failure. This is an example of similarity – a 50-year-old lady who is very wheezy with clear lung fields on the X-ray. This is also an example of the fact that diseases vary far more in their symptoms and signs in real life than those described in textbooks. On the basis of probability, a 50-year-old lady with type 2 diabetes, angina and hypertension who has never smoked is more likely to have heart failure as a cause of breathlessness than chronic obstructive pulmonary disease. Asthma is possible, but it would have to be severe to have not responded to treatment and the clinical findings do not support this. This case illustrates the value of probabilities, a data bank of previous clinical experience and that response to treatment (or not) is sometimes a way of making a diagnosis.

References

1. Modernising Medical Careers. www.mmc.nhs.uk
2. Eva K. What every teacher needs to know about clinical reasoning. *Medical Education* 2004; **39**: 98–106.

3. Hampton JR, Harrison MJG, Mitchell JRA *et al.* Relative contributions of history taking, physical examination, and laboratory investigations to diagnosis and management of medical outpatients. *British Medical Journal* 1975; **2**: 486–489.

4. Kirch W and Schafii C. Misdiagnosis at a university hospital in 4 medical eras. *Medicine (Baltimore)* 1996; **75**: 29–40.

5. Wray NP and Friedland JA. Detection and correction of house staff error in physical diagnosis. *Journal of the American Medical Association* 1983; **249**: 1035–1037.

6. Fletcher J and Fox R. Commentary: pattern recognition versus Bayesian approach for diagnosis in primary care. *British Medical Journal* 2006; **332**: 646.

7. Sox HC. Probability theory and the interpretation of diagnostic tests. In: Harold Sox (ed.). *Common Diagnostic Tests. Use and Interpretation,* 2nd edn. American College of Physicians, Philadelphia, 1990.

8. Doctors in Society. Medical professionalism in a changing world. Report of a working party of the Royal College of Physicians Dec 2005. *Clinical Medicine* 2005; **5(6) Suppl 1**: S1–S40.

9. PIOPED Investigators. Value of ventilation–perfusion scan in acute pulmonary embolism: results of the prospective investigation of pulmonary embolism diagnosis (PIOPED). *Journal of the American Medical Association* 1990; **263**: 2753–2759.

10. Klein Gary. *Sources of Power. How People Make Decisions.* MIT Press, Cambridge, MA, 1998.

11. Russo JE and Schoemaker PJH. *Winning Decisions: How to Make the Right Decision the First Time.* Piatkus, London, 2002.

12. Klein JG. Five pitfalls in decisions about diagnosis and prescribing. *British Medical Journal* 2005; **330**: 781–783.

Further resources

• Black ER, Bordley DR, Tape TG and Panzer RJ (eds). *Diagnostic Strategies for Common Medical Problems,* 2nd edn. American College of Physicians – American Society of Internal Medicine, Philadelphia, 1999.

• Kassirer JP and Kopelman RI. *Learning Clinical Reasoning.* Lippincott, Williams and Wilkins, Baltimore, 1991.

CHAPTER 5

Communication with colleagues

By the end of this chapter you will be able to:

• Understand how personality type affects the way we communicate
• Create understanding in teams and use 'netiquette'
• Know what makes a good leader
• Communicate clearly in clinical emergencies

People prefer to communicate in different ways, without realising. Sometimes these differences are a source of misunderstanding or irritation. Think about how you like to be served in a high street television store. Do you appreciate friendly assistants or do you avoid them? Is it more important to you that they know what they are talking about, or that they serve you with a personal touch? Do you buy your electrical goods on the Internet to avoid high street stores altogether? Asking this question of a group is very revealing, as all of us have very different preferences.

Personality type

Personality type influences the way people prefer to absorb information, make decisions and communicate. Understanding personality type can be helpful in understanding one's own preferences, strengths and weaknesses. In turn, this can improve understanding and communication between doctors and patients and between colleagues. There are different models of personality type, but one widely used and validated personality type indicator is the Myers-Briggs® system. Research using Myers-Briggs® suggests that personality type can have a significant bearing on student learning and doctor–patient communication, as well as working in teams [1].

In the Myers-Briggs® personality type indicator (MBTI), four basic aspects of personality are described [2]:

1 Introversion or extraversion (how you energise)
2 Sensing or intuition (how you take in information)
3 Thinking or feeling (how you make decisions)
4 Judging or perceiving (how you organise your life).

Introversion and extraversion

Introverts are not necessarily quiet people. They are very aware of their inner world and like to ponder and reflect. If they talk about something, they have probably thought about it first and need to do so without interruption. Conversations with introverts often include pauses and they can seem hard to get to know. Extroverts relate more to their outer world and prefer inter-action. They are more aware of people around them and more likely to greet people and interact in the workplace. Extraverts tend to think out loud and can be easy to talk to. Conversations with extraverts often include interruptions.

Sensing and intuition

People with a sensing preference see details and focus on the present and prac-ticalities. They want to know if something has been tested first, like to proceed step by step and like information to be precise and detailed. They prefer to do something rather than think about it. People with an intuitive preference focus more on the big picture and possibilities. They ask the question 'why' (rather than 'what' and 'how') and prefer the 'bottom-line' rather than a detailed description. They dislike 'boring details' and tend to think about several things at once.

Thinking and feeling

Thinking types make decisions based on objective analysis and tend to be task-orientated. Thinkers may appear (incorrectly) as if they have few emotions because they can discuss difficult subjects in a matter-of-fact way. They value competence highly. Feeling types make decisions based on values and tend to be people-orientated. They are more likely to express appre-ciation or thanks. They may find it extremely stressful if they have to tackle a difficult colleague about his behaviour. They value relationships highly.

Judging and perceiving

Judging and perceiving relate to how people organise their lives. Judging types make lists, plan ahead and enjoy completing tasks. They want to make deci-sions quickly. Perceivers 'go with the flow', live in the present, are flexible and dislike being rushed into making decisions.

You might have an idea which preferences you have. Overall there are 16 different combinations of Myers-Briggs® personality types. Personality type has been compared to right- or left-handedness; all of us use both hands but we naturally prefer one over the other. If we are aware of our own prefer-ences, strengths and weaknesses, it can help us to communicate better. Most complaints against doctors are related to poor communication rather than clinical incompetence [3].

In terms of communication, sensing/intuition and thinking/feeling are the aspects of personality type which are most important:

- A sensing and thinking person prefers practical facts, specifics, logical presentation and written information.
- A sensing and feeling person prefers practical facts but with a personal touch, friendliness and examples where others have experienced the subject under discussion.
- An intuitive and thinking person prefers competence, getting to the point, options and people who listen before giving advice.
- An intuitive and feeling person prefers an overview without too many details but with a personal touch and friendliness.

One study found that doctors were more likely to have intuitive and thinking personality types than the general population, illustrated in Fig. 5.1 [4]. This also has implications for inter-disciplinary communication (see Box 5.1).

It is easy to see how communication difficulties can arise at work if people do not understand that others are simply different. People can offend others without even realising. You may think others are antisocial, loud, emotional, uncaring, disorganised, obsessive, head-in-the-clouds, fussy and other negative terms when really what you are observing are other people's differences. For example, how do you like a patient to be referred to you over the telephone?

Personality type	Doctors (%)	Non-doctors (%)
Sensing and thinking	32.3	36.4
Sensing and feeling	17.2	40.1
Intuition and thinking	31.3	9.5
Intuition and feeling	19.2	14.0

Figure 5.1 Personality type of doctors compared with non-doctors.

Box 5.1 Inter-disciplinary communication

Clack *et al.* showed that most male doctors (and a higher proportion of female doctors than the general population) had a thinking preference whereas most nurses had a feeling preference [4]. This can have important implications for communication. In addition, differences in medical and nursing training lead to different ways of thinking and even a different culture. The first step is to realise these differences exist so that communication can be improved within the healthcare team. Can you think what these differences are?

Box 5.2 'Netiquette'

Netiquette is using technology effectively to communicate with others personally and professionally with knowledge, understanding and courtesy. E-mail communication can easily be misunderstood because most communication relies on visual cues. When using e-mail to communicate, the following things are important:

- Keep e-mails short and simple. Long e-mails are unlikely to be read
- Never send an e-mail in anger and do not use sarcasm
- If the subject matter is important, contentious or confusing, telephoning or arranging a meeting is a much more effective way to get things sorted out
- E-mails can appear unintentionally unfriendly. Adding occasional exclamation marks or emoticons (e.g. ☺) can help
- E-mails still require proper spelling and grammar. Remember to politely greet and sign off. Avoid capital letters as these are hard to read
- Check who the e-mail is being sent to – do you really need to 'reply to all'?
- Respond to e-mails promptly
- Do not forward e-mails without a comment even if it is only 'for your information'.

Resolving tensions in the workplace

Modern healthcare teams consist of individuals who are interdependent rather than independent of one another. Where there is courtesy, kindness, honesty and keeping commitments, there is trust. Where there is trust, communication does not have to be perfect, because people already understand one another.

There are some simple processes to creating greater understanding in teams [5]:
- Take time to understand what other people mean, their priorities and concerns before you express yours
- Small, everyday courtesies are very important
- Keep commitments
- Do not be afraid to apologise
- When faced with a problem, look creatively for a solution that can satisfy everyone involved, rather than choosing the obvious option in which someone loses out
- Realise that a team made up of diverse personality types and skills has greater potential than one made up of similar people.

E-mails can be a source of misunderstanding, which has led to the concept of 'netiquette', described in Box 5.2.

Leadership

Most doctors end up in positions of leadership. Leadership is knowing about people, rather than theory or structures [6]. We are all aware of how just one person can make a big difference to a department, whether for good or bad. Good leadership is characterised by the processes which create greater under-standing, listed above, and by pro-activity. Good leaders do not simply moan about the National Health Service (NHS); rather they focus on things which they can change and do something about it.

Delegation

In medicine, delegation is commonplace (see Box 5.3). Trainee doctors work with a qualified doctor who takes overall responsibility for the medical care of the patient.

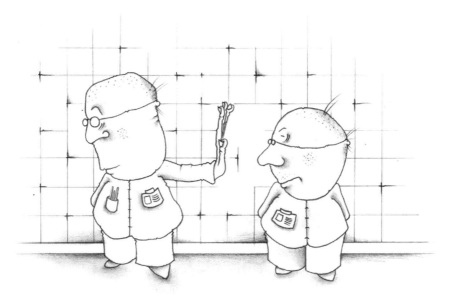

Communicating with colleagues.

Box 5.3 Delegation in practice

An senior house officer (SHO) was used to doing all the ward work and was unable to adapt to having a house officer on the ward. Instead of letting the house office organise tests, chase results and respond to requests from the nursing staff, the SHO did all of this himself. As a result, the house officer had no role on the ward. He switched off, felt under-valued and did not feel he was learning anything. In response to this, the SHO felt he had to do even more.

Delegation is actually a skill. To delegate properly, you need to [5]:
- Ensure a clear, shared understanding of the desired results
- Identify essential boundaries in which the individual has to operate and spell out anything he cannot do
- Identify what resources are available
- Describe the accountability structure
- Describe the benefits or consequences to the individual, team or organisation.

Many junior doctors start a new job without their role or what is expected of them being clearly communicated. If they perform poorly, is this a problem with the doctor, or with communication and leadership?

Statements of intent

Another important aspect of leadership is the fact that a team can only work together towards a common goal if everyone understands what that goal is. Communicating intent has been studied in the military and other organisations [7]. When people are told what to do without understanding why, they are less able to improvise or act independently and may assume things incorrectly. Communicating intent promotes shared understanding, independence and improvisation. When you communicate intent:
- There is less need for clarifications
- Problems are anticipated in advance
- People can react to circumstances 'on the ground' without having to get permission first
- People can think and plan ahead
- Team members can recognise and take opportunities.

The longer a team has been working together, the easier it becomes to anticipate what the person in charge would want. This poses a problem for doctors in training, who frequently move from team to team, so statements of intent are particularly relevant (see Box 5.4). Statements of intent are important at the start of a new job, before a significant task (e.g. the start of a theatre list), when delegating or when briefing a team. The statement should include [8]:
- This is what I think we face (big picture)
- This is what I think we should do (objectives, plan of action)
- This is why (rationale)
- This is what we need keep our eye on (key decisions, pitfalls)
- Now, talk to me (discussion, questions).

A good statement of intent is as short as possible, so that the main message is not obscured.

Communication in clinical emergencies

Communication in clinical emergencies has to be clear. For example, clear leadership and communication within trauma teams have a significant impact on patient care. Teamwork and patient safety are discussed further in Chapter 19. Junior doctors spend a significant amount of time describing clinical situations

Box 5.4 Statements of intent: clear and not so clear

At the start of a week of nights, the specialist registrar (SpR) calls the entire team (three SHOs and two house officers) together for a statement of intent. He states that they will work together as a team, gathers information on the current workload and patients waiting to be seen, describes each person's roles and responsibilities, explains that the team will have regular breaks together in order to get refreshed and discuss workload, explains why this is important (so no one feels isolated or is overworked whilst others have nothing to do) and describes situations of which he needs to be informed. The team has a discussion to clarify certain points before starting work. The result is a team that works well together, learns together and has a good week of nights.

An SHO called the SpR about an extremely agitated alcoholic patient who required sedation. The SpR asked the SHO to draw up a certain intravenous dose of midazolam and added 'I am on my way'. The SpR intended to give the drug herself when she arrived and intended to titrate the dose to the response of the patient. The SHO thought the SpR meant for her to give the drug and did so. The patient was unconscious by the time the SpR arrived.

to more experienced colleagues over the telephone, or asking for help in an emergency. A simple system for how to communicate when asking for help in an emergency is described in our companion book *Essential Guide to Acute Care* [9]:
- State where you are and your request (e.g. 'Can you come to …')
- Give a brief history (e.g. 'New admission with asthma')
- Describe the vital signs (pulse, blood pressure, respiratory rate, oxygen therapy and saturations, conscious level and urine output if relevant).

Further details can follow if needed and requested. Summarising the current vital signs is the main way of giving the listener a sense of how urgent the situation is. It is also important to communicate clearly what help is required. In other words, do not simply tell a story, state what you want from the other person; for example, 'Can you come now?', 'I am asking for advice' or 'Just to let you know'.

Key points: Communicating with colleagues

- Our personality type affects the way we communicate.
- Understanding personality type can help you understand your own preferences, strengths and weaknesses and communication in teams.
- Teams consist of interdependent individuals and there are important processes which help a team to work well together.
- Leadership is about understanding people rather than theory or structures.
- Leaders need to be able to communicate clearly and explicitly.
- In an emergency, clear communication is particularly important.

Exercises

- Describe any communication mishaps you have experienced which were probably related to personality type.
- With a group of others, discuss how you would like your doctor to break bad news to you – what aspects are particularly important? Are all members of the group the same?
- Think of the last patient you saw – how did he talk, what kind of questions did he ask, how did he decide things, how did he relate to you as a person? Can you identify what personality type he might have been? How could you tailor your consultation style in response to this?
- Describe situations in the workplace where delegation could be done better.
- Describe situations in the workplace where clear statements of intent could improve patient care.

References

1. Allen J and Brock SA. *Health Care Communication Using Personality Type. Patients Are Different!* Routledge, New York, 2000.
2. Myers IB, revised by Kirkby LK and Myers KD. *An Introduction to Type*, 6th edn. Consulting Psychologists Press, Palo Alto, CA, 1998.
3. Meryn S. Improving doctor–patient communications: not an option but a necessity. *British Medical Journal* 1997; **316**: 1922.
4. Clack G, Allen J, Cooper D and O Head J. Personality differences between doctors and their patients: implications for the teaching of communication skills. *Medical Education* 2004; **38**: 177–186.
5. Steven Covey. *The 7 Habits of Highly Effective People*. Simon & Schuster, London, 1989.
6. Steven Covey. *The 8th Habit. From Effectiveness to Greatness*. Simon & Schuster, London, 2004.
7. Klein G. Sources of power. *How People Make Decisions*. MIT Press, Cambridge, MA, 1998.
8. Weick KE. Managerial thought in the context of action. In: Srivastva S, ed. *The Executive Mind*. Jossey-Bass, San Francisco, CA, 1983.
9. Cooper NA, Forrest K and Cramp P. *Essential Guide to Acute Care*, 2nd edn. Blackwell, London, 2006.

Further resources

- Cooper NA and Forrest KA. Leadership and teamwork. *BMJ Career Focus* 2006; **332**: 46–47.
- Houghton A. The importance of having all types in a workforce. *BMJ Career Focus* 2005; **330**: 56–57.
- Houghton A and Allen J. Doctor–patient communication. *BMJ Career Focus* 2005; **330**: 36–37.
- Pelley JW, Delley BK and Smith LA (illustrator). Success types for medical students. A programme for improving academic performance. Texas Tech Univ Extended Studies, 1997. ISBN 0 9665 0490 9.
- The Myers-Briggs Foundation. www.myersbriggs.org.

CHAPTER 6
Medical records

By the end of this chapter you will be able to:

- Write in medical records appropriately
- Know what to write in medical records
- Understand the legal issues regarding medical records

Medical records are a key component of safe patient care. They are used to keep yourself and colleagues well informed about patients, for audit, coding and as a medico-legal document. Every hospital has its own guidance on medical records and national guidelines have existed for some time [1–3]. Yet poor medical records are commonplace. The term 'medical records' covers:

- Hand-written notes
- Discharge advice notes (or 'TTOs' – to take out)
- Letters
- Request and referral forms
- Computerised records
- Test results and images.

The General Medical Council (GMC) states that doctors should 'keep clear, accurate, legible and contemporaneous patient records which report the relevant clinical findings, decisions made, information given to patients [and relatives] and any treatment prescribed [1].' In legal terms, the interpretation of medical records is very simple: if it is not written down, it did not happen.

Hand-written notes

All hand-written records should be made in black ink. Other colours do not photocopy well when medico-legal reports are being prepared. The patient should be identified at the top of each page by name and unique identifier (hospital number). Before each entry, you should print your name, grade, date and time. For example:

1-2-06   Smith (SHO) 1800hrs

If you are writing for someone else you should make this clear by writing the doctor's name, not just 'consultant' or 'SpR (specialist registrar) ward round'.

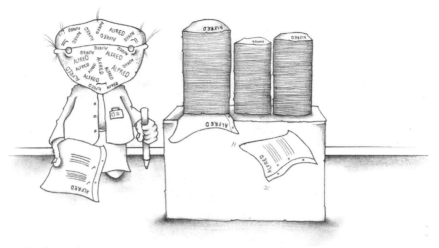

Medical records.

All doctors follow a standard structure when seeing a patient for the first time. The 'clerk-in' has been ingrained since medical school. However, what is not ingrained is how be clear about your management plan and how to write what you *think* as well as what you observe and do. The notes should make it easy for other members of the healthcare team to understand what is going on, what tests have been requested and why. At the end of the clerk-in, you should write a summary and a plan – and tick tests you have organised to make it clear to others what has been done. Sign your entry at the end.

When a patient has already been clerked in, subsequent entries should still detail history, examination, findings, plan, progress, information given and so on. Again, try and summarise what the team *thinks* is going on rather than just your observations and actions. Some people find the acronym 'SOAP' useful in structuring their notes:

S: subjective or patient symptoms

O: objective or clinical findings

A: assessment (including information given)

P: plan

An example of the 'SOAP' system is shown in Box 6.1.

All hospital inpatients should have a daily entry in their notes. Notes should be:

- Clear to everyone who reads them
- Accurate
- Legible
- Contemporaneous – written as soon as possible after the event
- Objective (personal, complaining or offensive comments are not appropriate)
- Original. A mistaken entry should be corrected with a single line through it with a signed, dated explanatory note. You must not alter an entry or disguise an addition

Box 6.1 An example of the SOAP system

1-2-06	SMITH (SHO) 1800hrs
S:	Asked to review patient re: sudden breathlessness
O:	Alert
	Sweating $++$
	RR 30/min
	Pulse 120/min regular
	SpO_2 86% on air
	BP 180/90
	Wheeze and widespread crackles throughout both lungs
A:	Acute left ventricular failure
P:	Sit patient up ✓
	15 l/min O_2 reservoir bag ✓
	5 mg nebulised salbutamol ✓
	80 mg i.v. frusemide ✓
	Portable chest X-ray ✓
	ECG done – shows ST elevation
	300 mg aspirin (chewed) ✓
	Cardiology team contacted and transfer to
	coronary care unit arranged ✓
	Patient much improved after i.v. frusemide
	Explained 'having a heart attack' and need for transfer

- Abbreviation free. Each hospital has a short list of authorised abbreviations, for example BP, temp and RR (blood pressure, temperature and respiratory rate).

Discharge advice notes or TTOs

These are the short letters that patients take away after discharge from hospital, with the date of admission and discharge, diagnosis and new medication list. They are often hand-written and a ballpoint pen should be used. Audits of such letters show that the information given is often of poor quality.

Imagine you are the general practitioner (GP) who has been asked to see the patient a few days after discharge from hospital. No formal discharge summary has been received. The TTO has to contain everything the GP needs to know about the admission. For example, 'chest pain no myocardial infarction (MI)' is meaningless. So is 'collapse', 'abdominal pain' or 'swollen leg no DVT (deep vein thrombosis)'. The GP will be asking himself, 'What was the working diagnosis? What were the medication changes and why? Which team was looking after the patient and is any follow-up arranged?'

A good discharge advice note has a concise but comprehensive diagnosis list. TTOs are held by patients and their relatives, so ensure they know about any diagnosis you write. The note should be clear and legible, with medications prescribed in block capital letters. Always check with your senior on the ward round what the final diagnosis is, as writing the initial rather than the final diagnosis can lead to all sorts of problems later.

Letters

Discharge summaries and clinic letters are the most commonly dictated letters by doctors. The patient's name and unique identifier (hospital number) should be clearly dictated at the start of each letter. Letters should *always* start with a comprehensive problem or diagnosis list. This makes subsequent patient care much easier.

Letters serve two purposes:

1 Information to the GP. GPs prefer concise letters with problem lists.
2 Information for future hospital visits. In some specialities, the first letter may contain a lot of detail about history, social circumstances and functional abilities.

If a patient is being discharged to a new residential or nursing home, it is vital that a letter is sent to 'the attending doctor' at the home on the day of discharge. The patient will probably have a new GP, have a complex medical background and the new home will have limited information about the patient unless you provide it. Where the patient has the capacity to do so, you should get consent for this. An outline of a discharge or clinic letter is shown in Box 6.2. The Department of Health guidelines on copying letters to patients are described in Box 6.3.

Doctors have the responsibility to check everything written in their name. You must check and sign all dictated letters.

Request and referral forms

The key to writing request and referral forms is to *ask a question*. Why do I want this test? Why do I want this specialist consultation? If you do not ask a specific question, you will not get a specific answer. For example, if you suspect pancreatic cancer in a patient but the pancreas was obscured by bowel gas on ultrasound, you should write specifically what you are looking for on the request form for a computerised tomography (CT) scan.

The Ionising Radiation (Medical Exposure) Regulations came into force in May 2000 as a result of a European directive [5]. These regulations mean that a doctor or other approved healthcare professional has a responsibility to justify the medical exposure involved in a test before it can be carried out. So for example, if you request a chest X-ray by writing 'unwell', it will be rejected by the radiology department. If you require a specialist test, it is often easier to discuss the case with the relevant expert.

Test reports must not be filed until a clinician has seen and signed them.

Box 6.2 Outline for dictating discharge and clinic letters

Discharge letters	Clinic letters
Name and hospital number	Clinic date
Date of admission	Name and hospital number
Date of discharge	Diagnosis list
Diagnosis list	1. a
1. a	2. b
2. b	3. c, etc
3. c, etc	Any action for GP (including
Medications (and changes)	medication changes)
Allergies	Follow-up
Follow-up	Dear Doctor,
Any action for GP	(Include what you think about
Dear Doctor,	the possible diagnosis and where
(Brief summary)	you are heading in terms of
	management – this makes it easier
	for colleagues who see the patient
	after you)

Help the secretary and the reader by being concise. There is no need to dictate 'this 70-year-old man was admitted with a cough, breathlessness and fever and his test results showed raised white cells and right lower zone consolidation on the chest X-ray …' when you can say 'Mr X was admitted with pneumonia.'

Computerised records

For computerised records, including results servers, the computer must be secure. Monitors should face away from public view. Data must be password protected and printouts must be shredded after use. Detailed guidelines exist on the required security characteristics of computerised medical records, ensuring the integrity, accountability and confidentiality of the data.

The National Programme for IT in the NHS [6] is a Department of Health project which aims to bring modern computer systems to the NHS over the next 10 years and improve patient care and services. This includes:
• Connecting GP surgeries to hospitals
• Electronic booking service (choose and book)
• An electronic patient record
• Electronic prescribing and transmission of prescriptions
• Picture archiving and communications system (PACS)

Box 6.3 Copying letters to patients

The Department of Health guidelines state that, 'As a general rule and where patients agree, letters written by one health professional to another about a patient should be copied to the patient or, where appropriate, parent or legal guardian … letters that help to improve a patient's understanding of their health and the care they are receiving should be copied to them as of right. Where the patient is not legally responsible for their own care (for instance a young child or a child in care), letters should be copied to the person with legal responsibility, for instance a parent or guardian' [4].

Copying letters to carers can be important (even though they are not legal guardians) and this should be done with the patient's consent. If the patient does not have the capacity to consent to this, the doctor should use his own judgement in the best interests of the patient. Letters should not be copied if:

• The patient does not want it
• There is information about a third party who has not given consent
• There may be problems with confidentiality (e.g. a sensitive and private issue is discussed, and there is a chance that the letter may be opened by someone else)
• The clinician feels it would cause harm.

Copying letters to patients means that some thought is required when dictating. Use plain English, avoid phrases that may unintentionally offend, stick to the facts and adjust some terms slightly or use brackets (e.g. anterior MI (heart attack)). However, the main purpose of the letter is to transmit clinical information and clinical accuracy should not be compromised.

• Patient decision aids
• A secure clinical e-mail service.

Currently, clinical coding is the process whereby non-clinical staff read paper medical records and summarise a clinical episode by entering standardised codes into a database. This is how hospitals receive payment for the work they do. In the future, such data will be recorded by clinical staff at the point of care using the electronic patient record.

Access to medical records

Medical notes belong to the person entering data in them (the doctor) and the NHS Trust. The following people have the right of access to medical records:

• A competent patient
• Those with parental responsibility, if it is in the child's best interests and not against the wishes of a competent child

- Other health professionals looking after the patient
- Solicitors acting for the patient.

Those who do not have automatic access (e.g. relatives, police, insurance companies, other solicitors) can apply for access or a report with the patient's written consent or a Court Order.

A doctor can show a patient his medical records if the patient is competent, it is unlikely to cause harm and there is no entry related to a third party who has not given consent. Otherwise, patients may formally apply to see their medical records under the Data Protection Act 1998. They can either view their records or request a copy for a fee. Box 6.4 shows the procedure which should be followed in such cases.

Finally, it is *everyone's* responsibility to ensure that notes are correctly filed and maintained.

Box 6.4 Access to medical records

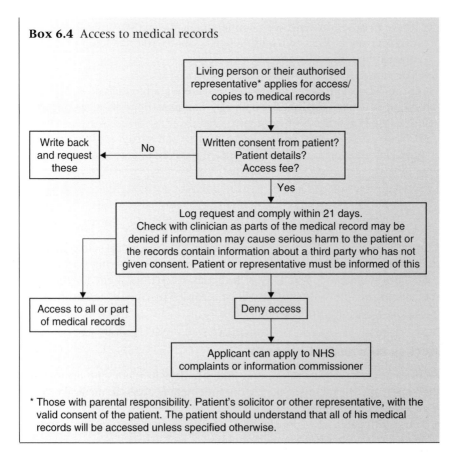

* Those with parental responsibility. Patient's solicitor or other representative, with the valid consent of the patient. The patient should understand that all of his medical records will be accessed unless specified otherwise.

> ## Key points: Medical records
>
> - Medical records should be clear, accurate, legible and contemporaneous.
> - All written entries must start with your name printed at the top, with your grade, date and time.
> - Record what you think as well as what you observe and do.
> - Tick tests you have organised to make it clear to others what has been done.
> - TTOs and letters should contain clear, concise problem lists rather than rambling narratives.
> - When writing referral or request forms, ask a question.
> - Department of Health guidelines are that letters should be routinely copied to patients.

Exercises

- Reflect on what you and colleagues write in the medical notes. Does it convey what you think as well as what you observe?
- Do you always begin a written entry by printing your name at the top?
- Practise writing concise but comprehensive problem lists on all correspondence
- Do you ask a question on request or referral forms, or do you just tell a story?

Self-assessment: Case histories

1 You are writing in the notes for the post-take ward round. A 40-year-old lady was admitted with epigastric pain which has resolved and was thought to be angina. The consultant and SpR have a conversation about the likelihood that this is in fact due to gallstones and the features that point to this. They explain this to the patient and discharge her. You write in the notes: 'patient is well, no further pain. Plan: discharge with outpatient abdo ultrasound'. The consultant looks at what you have written and says, 'That is not what we said.' What does he mean?

2 A patient on the ward wants to look through his medical notes. What is your reply?

3 Some relatives of an elderly lady want to look through her medical notes. One of them is a doctor. The other tells you he has 'power of attorney'. What is your reply?

4 The ward clerk asks you if she can file blood results before they have been signed. This would be easier for her, as she gets in at least 1 hour before the doctors each morning. What is your reply?

Self-assessment: Discussion

1 The patient was admitted with an initial diagnosis of angina. The subsequent entry in the notes does not explicitly state that the senior doctors think the

diagnosis is gallstones rather than angina. Actions rather than thoughts are recorded. A better entry would be: 'patient is well, no further pain. Clinical impression is gallstones rather than angina. No risk factors for ischaemic heart disease. Plan: discharge with outpatient abdo ultrasound.'

2 There is nothing to stop you from informally showing a patient your records if the patient is competent, it is unlikely to cause harm and there is no entry related to a third party who has not given consent. However, as a junior doctor you would be wise to refer this to your consultant or GP trainer and explain to the patient that he has a right to see your records, but you would like to inform your senior first, who may prefer to come and discuss any issues raised in the notes at the same time.

3 Relatives do not have an automatic right to access medical records, whether they are doctors or have any kind of power of attorney. They can apply for access with the written permission of the patient, if the patient has the capacity to give this (see Box 6.4).

4 All results must be seen and signed by a clinician before they are filed. This is to ensure that serious results which require action are not missed.

References

1. General Medical Council. *Good Medical Practice*, 2001. www.gmc-uk.org/ standards/ good.htm
2. Medical Defence Union. *Guidelines for Good Records*. www.the-mdu.com
3. Medical Protection Society. *Keeping Medical Records. A Complete Guide for Juniors*. London 2002. www.mps.org.uk
4. Department of Health. *Copying Letters to Patients. Good Practice Guidelines*. London 2003. www.dh.gov.uk
5. The Ionising Radiation (Medical Exposure) Regulations 2000 (together with notes on good practice). www.dh.gov.uk
6. www.connectingforhealth.nhs.uk

CHAPTER 7

Prioritising time

By the end of this chapter you will be able to:

- Prioritise according to clinical need
- Effectively organise your work for the day
- Deal with 'problem days'
- Understand that doctors are not perfect
- Plan for the longer term

The ability to manage time effectively comes more naturally to some people than others. But time management skills can be learned and are a vital part of the work of a doctor. During a normal day, a doctor needs to be able to prioritise:

- Clinical needs
- The needs of colleagues and family
- Time for important longer-term activities.

Clinical needs

A vital time management skill in medicine is the ability to prioritise according to the clinical need. For example, a case of cardiac chest pain is more urgent than a routine fluid prescription. A patient with seriously abnormal vital signs is more urgent than a patient who is relatively well with his chest infection. Certain conditions, for example, meningitis, ruptured aortic aneurysm and hyperkalaemia are urgent because they can cause a rapid deterioration. Good communication within teams is important so that prioritising can take place.

Triage is a common method of prioritising, used in the Emergency Department and in major incidents with multiple casualties. Surgical cases in the UK are prioritised according to National Confidential Enquiry in to Patient Outcome and Death (NCEPOD) criteria [1]:

- *Immediate*: life, limb or organ-saving interventions (to theatre within minutes)
- *Urgent*: acute onset or deterioration of a condition that threaten life, limb or organs (to theatre within a few hours)
- *Expedited*: early intervention for a condition that is not an immediate threat to life, limb or organs (to theatre within a few days)
- *Elective*: planned or booked surgical procedures (to theatre within weeks or months).

Using common terms to communicate the urgency of clinical need allows clear communication, appropriate clinical management and resource allocation.

Planning your day

In hospital practice, the day often starts with a ward round. After the ward round there will be a list of jobs to do, so make sure you write these down. These jobs need to be prioritised. One way to think of this is to apply the time management matrix, illustrated in Fig. 7.1.

Recognising the difference between important and urgent is a vital skill. This is because many people spend valuable time on urgent tasks, even though these might not be very important, and as a result neglect important tasks, even though these might not be very urgent. Being reactive in this way, rather than proactive, leads to stress and not necessarily achieving your goals.

Things that are both urgent and important are easy to recognise, for example, clinical emergencies and deadlines. However, it can be exhausting to always be in crisis mode. Time spent on important but not urgent tasks (the top right hand box in Fig. 7.1) helps to reduce crises and moves things forward rather than 'getting nowhere'. It may be that you have to change the way you personally work in order to spend more time on these tasks, or it may be that the system in which you work has to change (see Box 7.1).

The very nature of healthcare can mean that doctors are bombarded with information and tasks from all directions. This can be stressful, as most doctors want to do a good job. This kind of workload requires a system:

- At the start of the day, make a job list
- Clarify with your colleagues which tasks are more urgent or important than others
- Work through your job list in order of priority

	URGENT	NOT URGENT

IMPORTANT	**1**
	• Clinical emergencies
	• Imminent deadlines
	  (e.g. presentations,
	  assignments or patients
	  going to theatre)
		2
		• Reviewing daily blood results
		• Planning
		• Learning or revising for
		  examinations
		• Building relationships
		  (at home and at work)
		• Breaks and holidays

NOT IMPORTANT	**3**
	• Most interruptions
	• Some phone calls
	  and bleeps
	• Some meetings
		4
		• Watching television
		• Junk mail
		• Pleasant activities
		  (e.g. having a lie-in,
		  gossip over coffee)

Figure 7.1 Urgent and important tasks.

- Deal with constant interruptions by acknowledging the new task and adding it to your job list
- Break away from your work only to deal with clinically urgent matters or to grab an opportunity (e.g. speaking to relatives)
- Practise multi-tasking (e.g. can you do one job on the way to another to save time?)
- Accept the fact that there will always be work to do and you might never finish your job list
- Take regular breaks and do not miss food and drink
- Do not be afraid to ask for help if patient care requires it (see Box 7.2).

In hospital practice, taking time to hand over at the end of the day is particularly important. Take the last half an hour to ensure that all the non-urgent tasks such as fluid and warfarin prescriptions are written up, as this helps the on-call team. Ensure that sick patients or problems are handed over and every patient has a clear plan documented in the medical notes.

Box 7.1 Spending less time in crisis mode

A group of surgical house officers were exhausted from spending their whole working day in crisis mode and having no time to attend to important but not urgent matters. They felt stressed and wanted to deliver better clinical care. One of the problems was that so many patients needed to be clerked in before elective surgery on some days, that patients were signing consent forms on their trolleys, about to go theatre. The house officers decided to get together to formulate a plan they could present to their consultants. This included changing the pre-operative assessment clinic, re-allocating workload and introducing a bleep policy. As a result, the next group of house officers had a far less stressful experience.

Box 7.2 Prioritising on-call work

Ensure you get a hand over from the previous team so that you are aware of any sick patients and prioritise these. If you are covering the wards, visit each in turn. If there is no system where you work, ask your nursing colleagues to keep a job list for routine matters and to bleep you for urgent requests only. Tell them roughly when you will be back and try to be reliable. If you are covering an admission unit, see patients in the order of clinical priority, rather than in order of arrival. If you ever find yourself dealing with more than one emergency at the same time, get help.

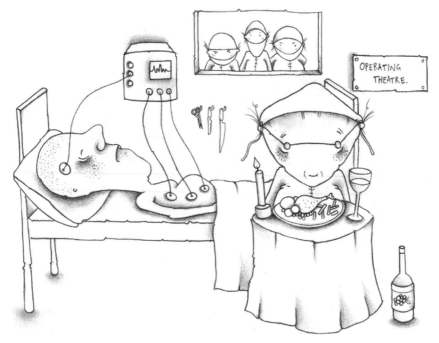

Prioritising time.

> **Box 7.3** Talking things through
>
> A general practitioner was having problems with Tuesdays. In the mornings her administration session was constantly interrupted by queries from the receptionist or practice manager. Most of these queries were not urgent. As a consequence, paperwork took longer than it should and she was always late for her visit to the local nursing home. At the nursing home she felt rushed and did not take the time she wanted to think through the patient's problems before dashing back (without lunch) for the evening surgery. On Monday evenings she was already feeling stressed about the next day. What do you think she could do about this?

Problem days

Some doctors find that they never seem to have enough time in the day, or that they have a recurring problem with one particular day. They recognise that the situation is stressful, but are unsure what to do about it. Talking this through with a trusted colleague can be a big help (see Box 7.3). Other people can sometimes see better how things might be able to change.

Doctors are not perfect

'No matter what measures are taken, doctors will sometime falter, and it is not reasonable to ask that we achieve perfection. What is reasonable is to ask that we never cease to aim for it' [2].

Doctors are expected to be:

- Organised
- Able to prioritise
- Flexible
- Punctual
- Available when on-call
- Hard working
- Able to recognise their own limitations.

This is quite a list and something to aim for, but a balance is required. People are not perfect, and unrealistic expectations can lead to stress and depression.

Some colleagues appear to be perfect. They are academically brilliant, play the violin in an orchestra, play squash to a national level and are the best husband and father. You struggle to make sure there is milk in the fridge, the bills are paid and your days end with you collapsing on the couch with a glass of wine, grateful that the day is over. The reality is that people who are successful in one area of their lives are often hopeless in another. Doctors are particularly poor at cultivating their home life and their own health. This is why pencilling in time for important but not urgent activities is so important.

Longer-term activities

As well as day-to-day organisation, people need to plan their time on a weekly basis [3]. If you do not timetable activities in your weekly diary they will not happen. We all have different roles, for example doctor, spouse, parent, friend and member of a choir. Think about your key roles and what your goals and ambitions are. The key to reducing stress and achieving your goals is to pencil in time for what you think are important activities. Use the time management matrix and divide activities into important/not important and urgent/not urgent.

Different people will put activities in different boxes. For example, one colleague thinks DIY is not urgent and not important, but she would not think the same if the bath were leaking and ruining the house. All activities can be important sometimes, even relaxing in front of the television, it just depends on whether you are avoiding more important activities.

An important way to reduce stress and realistically plan your time is to learn to say 'no' to requests. Practise a standard answer: 'Thanks. I would like to think about that and get back to you.' Do you have time to do this? Is there any advantage to you in making time to do this?

Although doctors get a sense of satisfaction and achievement from work, there are other important areas in which we need to achieve a healthy and enjoyable balance:

- Physical exercise (helps you feel and perform better)
- 'Spiritual' activities (e.g. religion, going for walks, reading novels)
- Relationships (which need nurturing).

Even the most flexible of personality types needs to learn to plan ahead to avoid stress, missed opportunities and burnout.

Exercises

- You are on-call. You have been referred the following patients: a 20-year-old man with a paracetamol overdose already on *n*-acetylcysteine treatment, a 30-year-old lady with diabetic ketoacidosis, an 80-year-old lady with a fall or a 50-year-old man with delirium tremens. How should you manage this workload?
- If your job is stressful and very busy, talk through the time management issues with a colleague for insight. Are there things about the way you work or the system which can be changed? What can you do about it?
- Do you spend enough time on important but not urgent activities?
- If you do not have a diary, buy one.
- Do you timetable non-medical priorities into your week?

References

1. *National Confidential Enquiry in to Patient Outcome and Death (NCEPOD)*. www.ncepod.org.uk
2. Gawande A. *Complications. A Surgeon's Notes on an Imperfect Science*. Profile Books, Croydon, 2003.
3. Covey S. *The 7 Habits of Highly Effective People*. Simon and Schuster, London, 1989.

PART II

Legal and Ethical Issues in Healthcare

CHAPTER 8

Capacity and consent

By the end of this chapter you will be able to:

- Assess capacity
- Know about the Mental Capacity Act 2005
- Understand the principles of consent
- Access legal advice when needed

All legal references in this chapter refer to the current law in England, Wales and Northern Ireland. Although most of the principles discussed here are relevant to the whole of the UK, readers working in Scotland should be aware that significant differences exist there.

Capacity

A medical procedure – in legal terms an examination, test or intervention – should only be carried out with the consent of the patient. For consent to be valid the patient must:

- Have the capacity to give or withhold consent
- Be given sufficient information so that he or she understands in broad terms the nature of the procedure, its likely effects and risks, the likelihood of success and any alternatives.

Box 8.1 Case history

An 80-year-old lady with dementia and agitated depression attended the chest clinic because of slight breathlessness which had been noted by her carers. Her chest X-ray showed what was likely to be lung cancer. The specialist registrar (SpR) did not feel that further investigation or treatment would affect the outcome in this case, but after talking with her son over the telephone, decided to admit her for a bronchoscopy. As you arrive on the ward, you hear the patient shouting out that she wants to go home. A message has been left that 'the son will consent for the bronchoscopy'. How do you proceed?

Capacity is a legal term and refers to a person's ability to do something, or make a decision which may have legal consequences. Capacity is an important principle in law, ensuring the right to autonomy. The English Courts have confirmed that: 'A man or woman of full age and sound understanding may choose to reject medical advice and medical or surgical treatment either partially or in its entirety. A decision to refuse medical treatment by a patient capable of making the decision does not have to be sensible, rational or well considered [1]'.

In law, there is a presumption that all adults have capacity, unless there is evidence to the contrary (which you have to document). To have capacity an individual must be able to:
- Understand and retain the information relevant to the decision
- Believe that information
- Weigh the information in the balance to arrive at a choice
- Communicate that decision in any form.

In some cases (e.g. advanced dementia or delirium) it may be obvious to you that a person does not have capacity to make a certain decision, which is why capacity is something that all healthcare professionals can assess. Lawyers and social workers also assess capacity – you do not need to call a psychiatrist to assess capacity except in cases which you find difficult.

The presence of dementia, mental illness or a learning disability does not necessarily mean lack of capacity. A person's capacity can be maximised by:
- Treatment of medical conditions which affect capacity
- Assessing the patient at his best time of day
- Making sure you can communicate effectively (e.g. use hearing aids, spectacles, privacy and time)

Capacity is not a general term. People have capacity *to make a certain decision*. A person may have the capacity to consent for a blood test or an X-ray, but not have the capacity to make a will or sell his house. In addition, capacity may fluctuate.

It is the personal responsibility of any healthcare professional proposing to examine, test or treat an individual to determine whether the patient has capacity at that time to give valid consent (Box 8.2).

If an adult temporarily or permanently lacks capacity to consent to a particular medical procedure, in England and Wales no other person (e.g. a relative)

Box 8.2 Case history

You go to assess the 80-year-old lady prior to her bronchoscopy and find that she is agitated and that it is impossible to have a conversation with her. The only thing you can determine is that she does not believe you are a doctor and this is not the hospital. It is obvious to you that this lady does not have the capacity to give or withhold consent to a bronchoscopy, since she appears unable at this moment to understand, retain, believe and weigh the relevant information, even in a limited form.

can consent on the patient's behalf. Doctors may still go ahead with the procedure on the legal basis of 'necessity'. This has two components:

1 There is a necessity to act.
2 The action is in the best interests of the person concerned (i.e. the expected benefits outweigh the burdens). Best interests is not limited to medical interests, this also refers to emotional, social, spiritual/religious and financial well-being, the person's right to liberty, quality of life, dignity and what is known about his preferences when he had capacity. This should be discussed by the team looking after the patient.

The role of relatives, therefore, is in helping you decide what is in the patient's best interests, because of their prior knowledge of the patient. In complex cases, or where the benefits and burdens of a medical procedure are finely balanced, a second opinion is recommended (Box 8.3).

The Courts have identified certain circumstances where referral should be made to them to decide on the lawfulness of a procedure in the case of incompetent adults, rather than being decided by the healthcare team:

- Sterilisation for contraceptive purposes
- Donation of regenerative tissue, for example bone marrow
- Withdrawal of nutrition and hydration in persistent vegetative states
- Where there is doubt as to the patient's capacity or best interests (after a proper assessment, further opinions and discussion between healthcare professionals).

Doctors are sometimes asked to assess capacity for outside agencies, for example a solicitor. Sometimes a patient may want to sign some papers and his solicitor will ask the ward doctor if the patient is 'capable' to do this. If you are ever asked to witness a legal document, be aware that as a doctor, you are also making a statement that the person has the capacity to sign that document, and therefore you have a duty to make an assessment first.

Box 8.3 Case history

You consider what would be in the best interests of the 80-year-old lady listed for bronchoscopy. You note that the test will not change the management of this lady's lung cancer and you feel a bronchoscopy would cause distress to her, and as a result may be technically difficult (and potentially more harmful) to perform. The ward sister agrees with you that:

- The patient lacks capacity to consent for this procedure
- Her son cannot give consent
- The procedure is not necessary and not in her best interests since it will not affect the outcome or management of her lung cancer and could cause harm.

You discuss the matter with a senior colleague and arrange to speak to the patient's son.

> **Key points: Capacity**
>
> - A medical procedure may only be carried out with the valid consent of the patient.
> - For consent to be valid a person must have capacity and be given sufficient information.
> - All adults are presumed to have capacity unless proven otherwise.
> - To have capacity you must be able to understand and retain, believe and weigh information.
> - Capacity is not a general term – it is specific to a particular decision.
> - Any doctor can assess capacity and a psychiatrist is only needed in difficult cases.
> - Capacity may fluctuate.
> - Relatives cannot give or withhold consent to medical treatment on behalf of an adult (except with a lasting power of attorney – see *further* on).

The Mental Capacity Act

This Act of Parliament became law on the 7 April 2005. The Adults with Incapacity Act (Scotland) 2000 offers similar provision, although the procedures and the names of Courts are different. For the first time in England and Wales, adults may make healthcare decisions on behalf of another adult who lacks capacity in certain circumstances if they:
- Have a lasting power of attorney
- Are an appointed Court of Protection deputy.

You may already of heard of enduring power of attorney (EPA) – this is where an adult with capacity can appoint another to deal with his property and affairs in the event that he might lack capacity in the future. When an EPA is organised, the 'donor' gives the legal right to one or more people (the attorneys) to manage his property and affairs, either immediately or in the future if he lacks capacity. Once a person becomes incapable, he can no longer appoint an EPA and a more convoluted and expensive process is required via the Court of Protection. An EPA does *not* allow a person to make decisions about healthcare on behalf of another.

'Lasting power of attorney' is a new concept, introduced by the Mental Capacity Act. An adult with capacity can appoint another, not only to deal with his property and affairs, but also to make decisions about personal welfare, which the Act defines as:
- Deciding where he is to live
- Deciding who can and cannot have contact with the person
- Giving or refusing consent to treatment
- Giving direction that another health professional should take over the care of the person.

The Act was designed, in part, for people to be able to plan ahead for a time when they may lose capacity. The Act is underpinned by five key principles:
1 The presumption of capacity unless proven otherwise

2 The right for people to be supported and helped to make their own decisions wherever possible
3 The right for people to make what might seem eccentric or unwise decisions
4 The principle of 'best interests' when a person lacks capacity
5 Anything done for or on behalf of people without capacity should be the least restrictive of their basic rights and freedoms.

A person's wishes can be put in to a written statement in advance, which must be considered in any decision making. This includes decisions to refuse treatment in certain situations (see Chapter 15). The Act also sets out guidance on *how* decisions should be made by the attorney or deputy and sets out certain limits.

Key points: Powers of attorney

- An *ordinary* power of attorney is something you can arrange via a solicitor if you go abroad for a year. It allows someone else to manage your property and affairs, but becomes invalid if you lose capacity.
- An *enduring* power of attorney remains in force if you lose capacity.
- A *lasting* power of attorney allows someone else to manage your property and affairs and make decisions about your personal welfare as well.

Principles of consent

Consent is required for medical procedures, research and teaching. Medical procedures range from major surgery to taking a blood test, giving an antibiotic or physiotherapy.

Consent can be express or implied. Express consent can be written, verbal or in sign language. Whether express or implied, consent has to be *valid*, which means given freely and with understanding. Performing a medical procedure without valid consent constitutes the offence of 'battery'.

Consent must be given freely, without undue influence from either family members or healthcare professionals. Patients must be given sufficient information so that they understand in broad terms the nature of the procedure, its likely effects and risks, the likelihood of success and any alternatives. Small but serious risks (e.g. death) and common risks need to be discussed.

Who is the best person to obtain consent? This depends on the procedure. For example, a competent nurse, doctor or student can quickly obtain verbal consent for a blood test. On the other hand, if an aortic valve replacement is being discussed with a 75 year old, an expert should spend time going through the procedure, its benefits and risks, with the patient and perhaps his family. Consent can be obtained as an outpatient before the procedure. Patients may need time to mull over information about major surgery before coming to a decision. Information can be provided by leaflets, video or by other members of the healthcare team. Consent is sometimes a *process*.

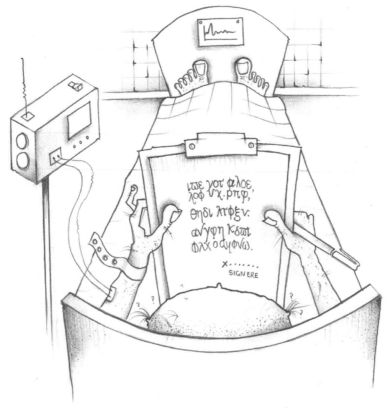

Consent.

There are many routine procedures, for example gastroscopy, where junior doctors may obtain consent provided they are competent to do so (i.e. know what the procedure involves and why it is being proposed, its effects, serious and common risks) and are able to do a basic assessment of capacity. However, a junior doctor should know the limits of his or her competence in obtaining consent and seek advice and training if needed.

What constitutes sufficient information? In 1985, the House of Lords decided in the Sidaway case that the legal standard to be used when deciding whether adequate information had been given should be the same as in negligence cases: a doctor would not be considered negligent in obtaining consent if their practice was the same as 'a responsible body of medical opinion in that field' (known as the *Bolam* test). However, they also stated that if certain information was so obviously necessary, it would be negligent not to provide it even if a responsible body of medical opinion would not have done so. So although the Bolam test remains influential, it should not be relied upon.

Box 8.4 National Health Service consent forms

There are four model consent forms used throughout the National Health Service (NHS):

- *Form 1*: patient agreement to investigation or treatment
- *Form 2*: parental agreement to investigation or treatment for a child or young person
- *Form 3*: patient/parental agreement to investigation or treatment (procedures where consciousness not impaired)
- *Form 4*: form for adults who are unable to consent for investigation or treatment.

It is also important to realise that the consent form itself is not a legal waiver. For example, if a person is not given sufficient information on which to base his or her decision, then the consent may not be valid even though the form has been signed. The consent form is not evidence of valid consent nor capacity to consent. Patients have the right to change their mind. In fact, signing a consent form is not even a legal requirement, except in certain circumstances (related to the Mental Health Act and the Human Fertilisation and Embryology Act). However, in practice, consent forms are used as a prompt and as legal evidence of consent (Box 8.4). For significant procedures, it is wise to document the information given and any other aspects of consent in the notes or a clinic letter.

When consent has been obtained in advance, you should check if the patient still consents before the procedure. There is no arbitrary time limit to consent as long as the circumstances have not changed.

Consent for people under the age of 18 years

Children (those under the age of 18 years) are entitled to consent to medical procedures as long as that consent is valid in the same way as for adults, that is given freely and with understanding. The same criteria for assessing capacity apply. However, there are important differences:

For children with capacity

- Children aged 16 years and above may consent to a medical procedure if they have capacity, without the additional consent of a person with parental responsibility. However, it is always good practice to involve the person's family, unless the patient wants to exclude them.
- Children aged below 16 years may also consent to a medical procedure if they have capacity (sufficient understanding and intelligence). This is known as 'Gillick competence' after a famous case in which a mother tried and failed to ensure that if her children under the age of 16 years were given contraception, she would have to give her consent. Children under the age

of 16 years, by their very nature, will have capacity to consent to some procedures but not to others. Although additional consent by a person with
parental responsibility is not required in the case of a Gillick competent
child, the child should be encouraged to involve his or her parents, unless
it would not be in the child's best interests to do so.

- Unlike adults, the refusal or withholding of consent by a competent person
  aged under 18 years may be over-ridden in certain circumstances either by
  a single person with parental responsibility or by the Court. The principles
  of 'necessity' and 'best interests' apply. The patient's confidentiality may
  have to be breached against his or her will.
- In an emergency, you may act to save the life of a person under the age of
  18 years even if the child or those with parental responsibility refuse (this
  is not the case with competent adults).
- Involve a senior doctor if you are obtaining consent from a person under
  the age of 16 years and there is disagreement between the child and those
  with parental responsibility, or the child asks you not to share information
  with them.

For children without capacity

- Consent may be given by a single person with parental responsibility or by
  the Court. The person with parental responsibility must have the capacity
  to consent, give it freely and with sufficient information.
- The Courts can over-rule a refusal by a person with parental responsibility.
  The welfare of the child is considered paramount.
- Consent by a single person with parental responsibility is valid, even if
  another refuses, although the Courts have said that important decisions
  should not be taken by one person with parental responsibility against the
  wishes of another – seek advice.

It is important to understand that 'parental responsibility' does not necessarily mean a parent. The Children Act 1989 sets out persons who may have
parental responsibility:

- The child's parents if married to each other at the time of conception or birth.
- The child's mother, but not the father if they were not married – unless the
  father has acquired parental responsibility through the Court, a parental
  responsibility agreement or the couple subsequently marry (or, as a result
  of new legislation, the father is on the birth certificate of a child born after
  1st December 2003).
- The child's legally appointed guardian.
- A person in whose favour the Court has made a residence order concern-
  ing the child.
- A Local Authority designated in a care order in respect of the child.
- A Local Authority or other authorised person who holds an emergency
  protection order in respect of the child.

There are certain situations where the healthcare team may disagree with a
person with parental responsibility, or doubt the competency of an adult to

withhold consent. Those with parental responsibility owe the child a duty to give or withhold consent in the best interests of the child and without regard to their own interests. If attempts at communication fail, an application can be made to the Court to decide. Applications to the Court can be made even in emergency situations (e.g. in the middle of the night to the on-call judge) although this is rare. Your hospital will have procedures in place for such an event and the consultant and medical director will be involved.

Key points: Consent

- For consent to be valid a person must have capacity, give it freely and have sufficient information.
- The validity of consent does not depend on the way in which it is given.
- An adult with capacity can withhold consent even if the reasons seem irrational and he will suffer harm or death as a result.
- Consent forms are used as a prompt and as legal evidence of consent.
- Obtaining consent may be delegated to competent junior doctors, but for complex or risky procedures should be obtained by an expert.
- Children with capacity may have their refusal over-ridden in certain circumstances by a person with parental responsibility or the Courts.
- The Courts hold that the welfare of children is paramount, and in certain circumstances those with parental responsibility may have their refusal over-ridden as well.
- In an emergency you may act to save the life of a child without consent from anyone (unlike adults, a child cannot refuse life-saving treatment).
- In complex cases, a senior doctor should be involved and remember that good communication is nearly always the key to resolving problems.

Exercises

- Have you ever witnessed relatives of an adult being asked to give consent?
- Describe situations where you have had to assess a person's capacity.
- Have you encountered any patient with a serious condition who refused treatment and had the capacity to do so? What happened?

Self-assessment: Case histories

1 An 80-year-old lady with severe dementia and behavioural problems is admitted to your ward because of hyperglycaemia. She has type 2 diabetes on insulin but is otherwise very well. She takes a long-acting insulin once a day. Each morning when the nurses go to give the insulin she folds her arms and refuses. How can you resolve this problem?

2 A 13-year-old boy is admitted to Accident and Emergency (A&E) accompanied by his 15-year-old girlfriend. She says he has 'taken some tablets' and it is likely that he has taken tricyclic antidepressant medication. He is twitchy, tachycardic and hypotensive. He is unresponsive. There is no contact number for his parents and he needs to be admitted to intensive care. What should you do?

3 A 20-year-old man is involved in a road traffic accident at 2 p.m. and has a ruptured spleen. He is hypotensive. As blood is on the way, his mother arrives and states that he is a Jehovah's Witness and must not be given blood products under any circumstances. What should you do next?

4 You rush to theatre with a 60-year-old man who has a ruptured aortic aneurysm. He is unresponsive since arriving in the A&E department but is normally fit and well. He is wheeled into theatre without a consent form and no one has been able to contact any relatives. Does this matter?

5 A 30-year-old lady is assessed in A&E for a paracetamol overdose. She says she took 50 tablets. Her husband is clearly very anxious about this, but she seems quite non-plussed. She does not want to be admitted to hospital and is very clear about that, despite her husband's protestations. What can you do about this?

Self-assessment: Discussion

1 Does the patient have the capacity to refuse her daily insulin? Can she understand and retain the information relevant to this decision, believe the information and weigh the information in order to arrive at her choice? If not, the insulin may be given against her wishes, in consultation with her relatives, in order to prevent life-threatening hyperglycaemia. The decision whether do this and the practicalities should be discussed by the whole healthcare team.

2 You do not need the consent of someone with parental responsibility to act in the best interests of a child in an emergency.

3 Jehovah's Witnesses are a religious group who believe that it is unacceptable to receive a blood transfusion. This includes fresh frozen plasma and platelets, although some individuals will accept immunoglobulin therapy or other blood derivatives so this should always be discussed. The patient is an adult and should be assumed to have capacity, unless there is evidence to the contrary. No one else can consent or withhold consent on his behalf. The patient should be given unbiased information regarding blood transfusion and you should ensure as far as you can that if he refuses, this is done without 'undue influence'. It is every capable adult's right to reject medical or surgical treatment either partially or in its entirety, in which case, you should explore all the possible alternatives available to him. The General Medical Council states in Duties of a Doctor: 'make sure that your personal beliefs do not prejudice your patients' care'. However, what if this patient is unconscious? You need to find out what evidence there is that the

patient would not want a blood transfusion in life-threatening circumstances and get expert help as soon as possible.

4 No.

5 This is a difficult assessment of capacity. Can this lady understand and retain the information relevant to her decision, believe the information and weigh the information in order to arrive at her choice? Is she suffering from a treatable mental illness (depression) which is clouding her judgement? A psychiatric assessment would be helpful here.

Reference

1. Sidaway vs Board of Governors of the Bethlem Royal Hospital and the Maudsley Hospital. Re S (Adult: Refusal of Treatment) (1993) Fam 123.

Further resources

- Assessment of mental capacity. *Guidance for Doctors and Lawyers*, 2nd edn. By the BMA and the Law Society, BMJ Books, London, 2004.
- The Association of Anaesthetists of Great Britain and Ireland. Report on managing anaesthesia for Jehovah's Witnesses. www.aagbi.org/pdf/7doc.pdf
- www.alzheimers.org.uk – information on how to arrange an enduring power of attorney from the Alzheimer's Society.
- www.bma.org.uk – members can access the ethics pages and get guidance on 'adults with incapacity medical treatment (Scotland) 2002' as well as a host of other general ethical and legal guidance.
- www.dh.gov.uk – information on the Mental Capacity Act from the Department of Health website. Guidelines on consent and model forms are also here.
- www.medicalprotection.org – useful information on a range of medico-legal issues by the Medical Protection Society.
- www.scotland.gov.uk/Topics/Justice/Civil/16360/5290 – information on the Adults with Incapacity Act (Scotland) 2000.
- www.the-mdu.com – useful information on a range of medico-legal issues by the Medical Defence Union.

CHAPTER 9

The Mental Health Act and common law

By the end of this chapter you will be able to:

- Know about the commonly used sections of the Mental Health Act
- Apply the Mental Health Act appropriately
- Understand when common law applies to the care of incompetent adults

The Mental Health Act (1983)

The law treats people with mental disorders differently in terms of:
- Compulsory detention and treatment in hospital
- Criminal cases
- The ability to deal in property and make contracts.

In law, a mental disorder is defined as 'a mental illness, arrested or incomplete development of the mind, psychopathic disorder or any other disorder or disability of the mind'. Drug or alcohol misuse or dependency is not included in this definition.

The Mental Health Act (1983) allows the relevant authorities to detain someone against his will in hospital to receive compulsory treatment for a mental illness. The Act is used when a person is at serious risk to himself or others. It allows for people to receive treatment against their will for *mental illness* or the causes of mental illness. It does not allow for people to be treated against their will for a separate *physical* condition (e.g. liver failure or severed hand tendons from an act of deliberate self-harm). The only exception where a physical condition may be treated under the Mental Health Act is in cases of anorexia nervosa where tube feeding may be authorised – here the weight loss is deemed to be an integral part of the mental illness.

The sections of the Mental Health Act that are most relevant to junior doctors are Sections 2–4 and 5(2):
- Section 2 allows compulsory admission for assessment and treatment for 28 days. An 'approved' social worker or the nearest relative can apply, and two doctors must provide recommendations. One of the doctors must be an approved specialist under Section 12 of the Act (often a consultant or

specialist registrar in psychiatry) and the other should ideally know the patient or also be approved, though this is not obligatory.

- Section 3 allows compulsory admission for assessment and treatment for up to 6 months. The same people are involved as above, though this time there is a requirement for the approved social worker to gain the consent of a relative.
- Section 4 is only occasionally used and is essentially the same as Section 2 although only one (approved) doctor is needed. It lasts for 72 hours and is usually turned into Section 2 as soon as possible.
- Section 5(2) allows for a patient in hospital for any reason to be detained for 72 hours if the doctor in charge of his treatment (e.g. consultant) or a deputy (e.g. specialist registrar) thinks that an application should be made for a proper assessment under another section. Section 5(2) does not allow treatment without consent, it merely allows detention and it only applies to hospital inpatients, not the Accident and Emergency (A&E) department.
- Registered mental health nurses can also detain patients who are hospital inpatients for up to 6 hours under Section 5(4), if they think that this is necessary for the safety of the patient and others, in the event that a doctor cannot attend immediately.

Sections 135 and 136 are used by police officers to remove a person with a mental disorder to a place of safety. A place of safety may be emergency social services accommodation, a care home, hospital, the police station or 'any other suitable place' – there are usually local policies about what constitutes a 'place of safety' and using the A&E department is usually avoided unless the person is physically unwell.

Medical and nursing staff are not *obliged* to restrain or contain people detained under the Mental Health Act. In fact, this could lead to physical harm coming to members of staff. Experienced staff are often able to 'talk down' mentally disturbed people. If you find yourself in a situation where a patient detained under the Mental Health Act becomes out of control and tries to leave, think of your own safety and that of your colleagues and other patients first. Let the patient leave if necessary. Call hospital security or the police, as they are better suited to deal with violent situations.

The common law

As mentioned before, the Mental Health Act applies to mental disorders, which excludes drug or alcohol misuse and unrelated physical illnesses. The Mental Health Act can in theory be applied to delirium and dementia, but treatment of these conditions is usually under common law.

The common law is used by healthcare professionals to detain or restrain incapacitous patients in order to ensure their safety and the safety of others. Only the minimum restraint necessary should be used. Restraint may be physical (e.g. holding a person or standing between him and the doorway) or pharmacological. An example might be in the case of delirium tremens, when a person withdrawing from alcohol and hallucinating is attempting to leave the ward by climbing out of the window. Such a person often has fluctuating concentration, and may be 'talked down' in the early stages, and offered a sedative such as a short-acting benzodiazepine. However, it may be necessary to restrain that person or give an injection of a benzodiazepine in his best interests, if he lacks the capacity to withhold consent to treatment.

Another example might be in the case of delirium due to infection in a person with dementia. You might find yourself with a patient who is paranoid and attempting to harm other patients or staff, or trying to leave the ward in the middle of a winter's night, wearing only a hospital nightie. Again, such people are often persuadable and restraint is a last resort, in their best interests and out of necessity. You must take care that you do not use restraint out of convenience, or because you are not experienced in dealing with delirious patients, or because you have misjudged someone's lack of capacity (e.g. the patient may be cantankerous and unwise rather than incapacitous). As a junior doctor, you should always involve a senior and ensure that you are able to justify your actions, including an assessment of capacity, in the medical notes.

In theory, the Mental Health Act could be used in cases of delirium to provide protection for the patient and treatment of any underlying physical illness *causing* the delirium. But it could not be used to treat an unrelated physical illness which is not affecting the person's mental state (e.g. alcoholic liver disease). Remember that Section 5(2), commonly used on general wards, is only a detention and not a treatment order. Therefore any treatment given to an incapacitous adult is given under common law and using Section 5(2) is therefore unnecessary. Fig. 9.1 outlines when treatment can be given against a person's will.

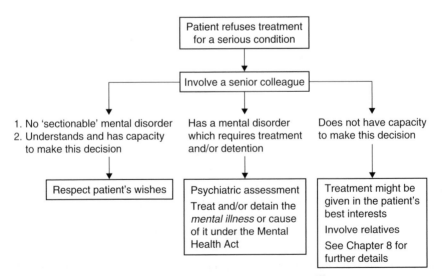

Figure 9.1 When treatment can be given against a person's will.

Dealing with violence and aggression

All junior doctors have access to violence and aggression training via local acute or mental health trusts. These courses help you learn how to defuse potentially violent situations and are particularly useful for healthcare staff working in A&E departments, medical admission units and in psychiatry. You can check the availability of these courses via your Trust Intranet, ward manager or general practice trainer. Intoxication is not a reasonable defence, so a person who is drunk in A&E who assaults a member of staff is still liable to prosecution. See the National Health Service (NHS) 'zero tolerance' campaign at www.nhs.uk/zerotolerance/intro.htm.

Key points: The Mental Health Act and common law

- The Mental Health Act allows the relevant authorities to detain someone against his will in hospital and receive compulsory treatment for a mental disorder.
- The Mental Health Act does not allow for a person to be treated against his will for an unrelated physical condition.
- Drug or alcohol misuse is not a mental disorder as defined by the Act.
- Section 5(2) of the Mental Health Act allows for any hospital inpatient to be detained for 72 hours if the consultant in charge of his treatment thinks that an assessment under the Mental Health Act is required. This only permits detention, not treatment.
- Hospital inpatients who are at risk of endangering themselves or others due to delirium can be managed using common law under a doctor's duty of care.

Exercises

- Have you ever experienced having to restrain a patient for their own safety or that of others? Describe the incident. Were you unclear about the legal issues at the time?

Self-assessment: Case histories

1 A 60-year-old man with a previous history of depressive illness has become steadily more unwell over the past 2 months. When his general practitioner visits him, the patient is slowed in his actions and expresses delusional beliefs about a hopeless future and has stopped looking after himself, his pet dog and his house. The patient will not eat solid food because 'it is poisoned' and thinks that the general practitioner is part of a plot to 'slowly rot his body'. He refuses to be assessed in hospital. Does the Mental Health Act apply here?

2 A 40-year-old man has attempted to sever his femoral artery to end his life. He is in the A&E resuscitation room. The patient is allowing someone to

apply pressure to the affected groin, but is unkempt and incoherent. He has a past history of chronic schizophrenia and is claiming to be an alien capable of supernatural regeneration. How does the Mental Health Act and Common Law apply to treatment of his injury?

3 An 85-year-old man develops post-operative delirium due to a combination of infection, pain and medication. At 1 a.m. he runs rampant around the surgical ward, grabbing the metal clipboards at the end of other patients' beds and throwing them at people. He spent some time as a prisoner of war in the Far East during World War II, and thinks he is in a concentration camp and that you are his guards. Despite attempts to orientate him, including a well-lit side room and the presence of his son, there is no reasoning with him. You feel that he has absolutely no idea what is going on, and that restraint is required in order to protect the patient and others from harm. Does the Mental Health Act apply here? What would be the best thing to do in this situation?

4 A 75-year-old man with dementia becomes agitated each evening on the ward. He is waiting for a place in a secure residential home. Each evening he wanders about, asking repeated questions and wanting to know what everyone is doing. He usually attempts to go home with a bag. He has already been assessed by a consultant psychiatrist who has agreed that the patient lacks capacity to decide on his future care due to dementia. In the mornings, when the patient is more lucid, he understands that he is waiting to go to a residential home. Does the Mental Health Act apply here? Can he be prevented from leaving the ward?

5 A 30-year-old man is admitted to hospital for treatment with intravenous *N*-acetylcysteine (Parvolex®) after taking 100 paracetamol tablets, staggered over 48 hours. He has now changed his mind about treatment and will not allow the second infusion to be started. The nurses also found some pieces of cut glass in the bedside locker, with which the patient attempted to cut his wrists. He also disconnected his drip and allowed himself to bleed before this was spotted by a member of staff. He says he is not having any hallucinations and does not seem delusional, but he does seem withdrawn and is behaving strangely. You decide to consult a psychiatrist on the matter. What does the Mental Health Act allow in terms of treatment for his paracetamol overdose?

Self-assessment: Discussion

1 Yes, Section 2 or 3 of the Mental Health Act would apply here.
2 In this case, the common law should be used, as the patient lacks capacity to refuse treatment for his severed femoral artery. The Mental Health Act would be used subsequently to ensure his safety and treat his mental illness.
3 The Mental Health Act need not apply here. This patient clearly lacks capacity and may be restrained under common law and duty of care, in his best interests. The minimum amount of physical and chemical restraint needed

Older patients with prior cognitive impairment, on psychoactive drugs with severe physical illness (or post-operative) are most at risk of delirium. Repeated reassurance and orientation, non-pharmacological sleep promotion, early mobilisation, providing visual/hearing aids and avoiding dehydration can prevent delirium[1].

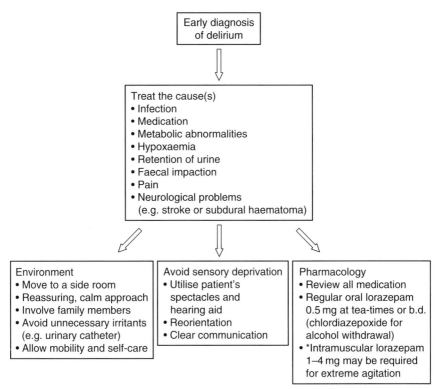

*Consult a senior first.
Around half of delirious patients have significant new cognitive impairment several weeks later.

Figure 9.2 Strategy for treating agitated delirium.

should be used, to allow you to look for and treat the underlying cause of his delirium (see Fig. 9.2). Hospital security can be called to help. The on-call psychiatrist can give advice even if the Mental Health Act is not required. Technically, Section 5(2) could be used to prevent him from leaving the ward, but you can still do that under common law, and any restraint and treatment *has* to be done under common law, so the Mental Health Act is unnecessary.

4 It would be most unusual for the Mental Health Act to be applied in this situation. It has already been agreed that the patient lacks capacity to decide his future care. In his lucid moments, he understands that he is waiting to go to a residential home. In the evenings, when he is more confused he can be prevented from leaving under common law and duty of care. This may

simply mean that the ward doors are locked, or that a member of staff persuades him to come back. Security or the police may be called to help if he manages to leave.

5 The Mental Health Act only allows for the assessment and treatment of his mental condition. Section 5(2) then 2 may be used here. The on-call psychiatric team should be involved. The Mental Health Act does not allow you to give N-acetylcysteine (Parvolex®) against a person's wishes, as this is treatment for a separate physical condition (liver failure). If the patient lacks the capacity to refuse treatment, it may be given under common law, but a careful assessment should be made of the patient's capacity by an experienced doctor. The patient may accept treatment with persuasion. Alternative treatments could be tried (e.g. methionine tablets).

Reference

1. Inouye SK, Bogardus Jr ST, Charpentier PA, Leo-Summers L *et al.* A multicomponent intervention to prevent delirium in hospitalised older patients. *New England Journal of Medicine* 1999; **340**: 669–676.

CHAPTER 10
Confidentiality

By the end of this chapter you will be able to:

- Understand what is meant by patient confidentiality
- Know the procedure for disclosing information to a third party
- Know under which circumstances confidentiality may be breached without consent

Confidentiality is the cornerstone of the doctor–patient relationship. Patients should feel that they can tell the doctor any information which would help in their care. The principle of patient confidentiality is found in:

- Medical ethics
- General Medical Council (GMC) standards
- Your contract of employment
- Access to Medical Reports Act 1988
- The Data Protection Act 1998
- Article 8 of the Human Rights Act 1998.

During a normal working day, confidentiality may be breached in several unintentional ways:

- During hand over of shifts
- Talking with colleagues in the lift
- Leaving the notes open on a desk
- Having a computer screen facing a public area
- Talking with a patient behind curtains.

It is the responsibility of every healthcare professional to take *reasonable* steps to ensure that patient confidentiality is protected.

Confidentiality applies to all personal information about patients (Box 10.1). However, patients tend to understand that information about them will be shared within their healthcare team or that their name will be included on a board on the ward, for example. Occasionally, patients speak in confidence to one member of the team and ask them not to disclose information which is highly relevant to their care. In these circumstances, you should explain beforehand that you cannot withhold relevant information from other key members of the team. Consent is required if personal information is to be shared with an outside agency (e.g. social services).

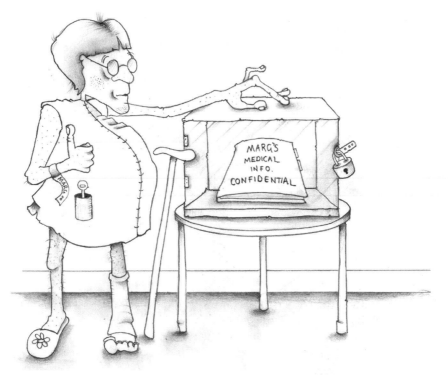

Medical confidentiality.

Box 10.1 'Caldicott guidelines'

These are guideines on releasing information about patients [1] and state that information (personal details, records and radiology) should be:
- Held securely and confidentially
- Obtained fairly and efficiently
- Recorded accurately and reliably
- Used effectively and ethically
- Shared appropriately and lawfully.

All members of staff working in healthcare, for example porters, kitchen staff and cleaners are bound by a duty of confidentiality, even if their contracts or professional bodies do not include it. Confidentiality applies even after death. Any disclosure must be justified and take into account the patient's previously expressed wishes. If a patient's confidentiality is breached without his consent, disciplinary, civil or criminal proceedings against the healthcare professional involved may result. There are exceptions to this, which will be discussed later.

Disclosing information to a third party

Patients can consent to their medical information being disclosed to a third party. In fact this is quite common for case reports in journals, insurance reports, Driver and Vehicle Licensing Agency (DVLA) reports and police statements. The consent should be in writing, and the patient should understand exactly what will be disclosed, to whom and for what purpose. You should ask the patient if he would like to see the report before it is sent.

Information is commonly shared with relatives or carers. It is good practice to make it part of your routine clerk-in to ask the patient who they are happy for the healthcare team to talk to. The consent to disclose information to relatives or carers is usually implied when a patient is seriously ill or lacks capacity to give consent. Patients often arrive in the outpatient department or general practitioner surgery with another person, implying that they are happy to share personal information, but you should always check this, particularly if you intend to discuss a sensitive matter.

If the healthcare team believes that a patient may be a victim of abuse, you may be obliged to disclose this information. This is discussed further in Chapter 13.

Police statements

Information to the police may not be given without consent except in the following circumstances:
- When the patient has assaulted you or your staff
- Under the Road Traffic Act, when the police can request the name and address of a driver who may be guilty of an offence, but not clinical information
- Under the Prevention of Terrorism Act, when there is a duty to disclose an act of terrorism or planned terrorism
- When disclosure may prevent a serious crime.

In these circumstances, you need only disclose relevant information.

Information to solicitors

Solicitors should provide evidence that the patient has consented to his medical details being disclosed. Check whether the request is from the patient's own solicitor or a solicitor acting for another party and that the patient understands the implications of disclosure.

Legal reports are protected by 'legal privilege' which means they should not be stored in a patient's medical notes where they can be accessed by other people and another legal team.

When confidentiality may be breached

Healthcare professionals have certain statutory obligations to report:
- A notifiable disease
- A birth at which they were present

- An accurate cause of death on a death certificate
- A termination of pregnancy which they have performed.

Confidentiality may also be breached by Court Order, or when doing so is essential to protect the patient or others from serious harm. This is referred to as 'the public interest'. The GMC has specific guidance on this, contained in the document 'Confidentiality: protecting and providing information' [2].

The GMC states that patient consent should be obtained where possible, but gives example where this may not be practical:

- When the patient lacks capacity to do so
- When it is an emergency and there is no time.

Examples of 'the public interest' might be if you know a person is still driving when a medical condition makes this dangerous to do so, or a person with a serious communicable disease is knowingly putting others at risk, or when a person informs you of his intention to abuse a child. In these kinds of situations get advice from your seniors and defence organisation.

Key points: Patient confidentiality

- Confidentiality is a cornerstone of the doctor–patient relationship.
- It is the duty of every healthcare professional to take reasonable steps to ensure that patient information is protected within the healthcare team.
- Make it a routine part of your clerk-in to ask patients who they are happy for you to share information with.
- Patient information may not be disclosed to a third party without consent except in certain circumstances.
- When patients do not have capacity or are seriously ill, their consent to disclose medical information to their next of kin is implied.
- Remember that good communication with relatives and carers is important.

Exercises

- Look at all the unintentional ways that confidentiality can be breached. Count how many times this happens in a normal working day and discuss how this issue could be addressed.

Case histories: Discussion

1 You receive a telephone call on the ward from a solicitor asking you to confirm that his client was an inpatient on your ward a few days ago. This is so that he can explain why his client missed a court appearance. What is your reply?

2 A relative telephones to make an appointment with the senior doctor. She is unhappy about the way her mother's condition has been managed and wants to discuss it. What is your reply?

3 You are working in Accident and Emergency (A&E) and have just treated a man with cuts to the side of his head. He smelt of alcohol and said he had been in a car accident. After the patient has left, the police arrive and ask for his name and address and details of what happened. What is your reply?

4 You are on the ward when a relative asks you for information about a patient. What is your reply?

5 You are treating a patient for a fracture of his fifth metacarpal in A&E who is agitated and talks constantly of returning home to 'finish off' his girlfriend. You are worried a serious assault might take place. What do you do?

Case histories: Discussion

1 Ask if the solicitor can fax a request on headed notepaper to the ward, with the signed consent of the patient, if possible. Or you could telephone the patient to ask permission to disclose this information. Tell the solicitor that you will call him back later.

2 Help to set up the appointment, then check with the patient that this is okay.

3 Under the Road Traffic Act you are obliged to give the name and address of a person who may have caused an offence, but you are not obliged to reveal any clinical information. The police can apply for a clinical report through official channels. However, if the patient told you he is about to drive home, you might want to reconsider what information you give to the police, in the public interest.

4 Check who the person is and ask whether the patient knows he or she has come to talk to you. Or ask the relative to wait a minute and go and ask the patient if it is okay. If the patient is seriously ill or lacks capacity to give consent to disclose medical information, it is assumed that they would want to share information with close relatives, except if they have previously expressed a view to the contrary.

5 Try and delay the patient in the A&E department whilst you discuss this with a senior. Is there evidence of mental illness? Should the police be informed? Very often in these situations there is no easy or right answer. You have to decide what is the best thing to do and be able to justify it based on the information available to you at the time.

References

1. Department of Health. The Caldicott Committee. *Report on the Review of Patient Identifiable Information*. Department of Health, London, December 1997.
2. www.gmc-uk.org/guidance/library/confidentiality.asp

CHAPTER 11

Death certification and the coroner

By the end of this chapter you will be able to:

- Complete a death certificate
- Know which deaths should be referred to the coroner
- Fill in a cremation form

The coroner system does not apply to Scotland and therefore any references to the coroner apply only to England, Wales and Northern Ireland. The Home Office has published a review: 'Reforming the Coroner and Death Certification Service: A Position Paper'[1], so changes to the system may take place in future.

Death certificates are essential for the following reasons. They are:

- A legal record of the fact of death, allowing the family to arrange disposal of the body and settle the estate of the deceased
- A means by which any 'unnatural' deaths can be investigated
- A vital source of epidemiological information.

The Births and Deaths Registration Act 1953 requires that all deaths must be registered by notifying the local Registrar of Births and Deaths within 5 days. A 'qualified informant' should do this, usually a relative. A medical certificate is required to register the cause of death and then burial or cremation is authorised. In England and Wales, 70% of deaths result in cremation and this requires first an application then a three-part medical certificate to be completed (unless the death has been referred to the coroner). The reason why further certificates or the authorisation of the coroner is required for cremation is because the 'evidence' as to the cause of death is about to be destroyed.

An accurate cause of death on the certificate is extremely important both epidemiologically and medico-legally. Audits show that junior doctors frequently write inaccurate death certificates, therefore, causes of death should always be discussed with a senior doctor first. The fact that a death has occurred is recorded in the medical notes. The death certificate records the cause of death 'to your best knowledge and belief'. Therefore, only a doctor who attended the deceased during his last illness can sign a death certificate.

An example of the first page of a death certificate is shown in Fig. 11.1. Details on a death certificate include:

- Details of the deceased
- Date and place of death

MEDICAL CERTIFICATE OF CAUSE OF DEATH

For use only by a registered medical practitioner who has been in attendance during the deceased's last illness

Name of deceased ....
Date of death as stated to me ....
Place of death ....
Last seen alive by me ....

Please circle the appropriate number or letter:

1. The certified cause of death takes account of information obtained from post-mortem
2. Information from post-mortem may be available later
3. Post-mortem not being held
4. I have reported this death to the coroner for further action (see overleaf)

a. Seen after death by me
b. Seen after death by another medical practitioner but not by me
c. Not seen after death by a medical practitioner

Cause of death

The condition thought to be the underlying cause of death should appear in the lowest completed line of part 1

	Approximate interval between onset and death (optional)
1(a) Disease or condition directly leading to death .... MYOCARDIAL INFARCTION (HEART ATTACK)	....
1(b) Other disease or condition, if any, leading to 1(a) .... ISCHAEMIC HEART DISEASE	....
1(c) Other disease or condition, if any, leading to 1(b)	....
2 Other significant conditions contributing to the death but not related to the disease or condition causing it .... DIABETES, CHRONIC RENAL FAILURE, OBESITY	....

The death may have been due to or contributed to by the employment followed at some time by the deceased (tick where applicable) ☐

Signature:
Qualifications as registered by the General Medical Council:
Residence (address):
Date:
For deaths in hospital, please give the name of the consultant responsible for the above named patient:

Figure 11.1 Example death certificate.

- Cause of death (1a–c and 2)
- Your details, including when you last saw the deceased alive.

On the other side of a death certificate there is a box to tick if the death has been referred to the coroner for any reason.

Which deaths need referral to the coroner

It is mandatory to notify the coroner if the death:
- Occurred within 24 hours of admission to hospital
- Is of unknown or uncertain cause
- Is related to, or within 24 hours of, surgery or anaesthesia
- May be related to a medical procedure or treatment
- May be a result of lack of medical care (if there is an allegation of medical mismanagement it is wise to report the death)
- Was related to an accident whenever it occurred (e.g. road traffic deaths, workplace deaths or a fall leading to a fractured neck of femur)
- Was due to self-neglect or neglect by others
- Was violent, unnatural (e.g. poisoning including acute alcohol intoxication) or suspicious
- Was related to an industrial disease (e.g. chronic obstructive pulmonary disease in an ex-miner)
- Was a suicide
- May have been due to an illegal abortion
- Occurred in, or shortly after, police or prison custody
- Occurred whilst the deceased was detained under the Mental Health Act
- Has any other usual or disturbing features to it.

The Registrar of Births and Deaths is also obliged by law to report deaths to the coroner where the deceased had not been seen by a doctor within 14 days of death or during his last illness, or where the deceased has not been seen by a doctor after death. It is an offence to bury or dispose of a body before the coroner makes enquiries or holds an inquest. It is also an offence to obstruct a coroner in his duty. If a death has been reported to the coroner the Registrar will be unable to register the death until the cause of death has been established, either by enquiry, post-mortem or inquest.

Out of 550,000 deaths in England and Wales per year 200,000 are referred to the coroner and 120,000 require a post-mortem. There are 20,000 inquests held each year. The role of the coroner (who is either legally or medically qualified) is to scrutinise reported deaths. In Scotland similar duties are performed by the procurator fiscal. If the death appears violent or unnatural an inquest must be held. If the death was sudden or unexpected but likely to be due to natural causes an inquest is not required. The coroner may order a post-mortem examination as part of his investigation.

A number of coroner's officers support the coroner, and these are the people doctors usually speak to over the telephone when reporting a death. Coroner's officers have usually trained as police officers and this must be remembered when using medical terms, even though most coroner's officers will be familiar with common terms. If an inquest is held (sometimes with a jury), the role of the coroner's court is not to establish liability but to establish the facts of how, when and where the death occurred. It will hopefully be a rare experience to have to attend an inquest, but if you do, contact your defence organisation who will provide you with valuable information.

Cause of death

The 'disease or condition directly leading to death' on a death certificate does not mean the *mode* of dying. For example, heart failure, cardiac arrest and septicaemia are not allowed on a death certificate as unqualified causes of death. Heart failure, cardiac arrest and septicaemia have many causes and are considered ways rather than causes of dying. However, you may write cardiac arrest as a cause of death if it is qualified as being due to ischaemic heart disease, for example.

Old age can only be given as a cause of death when all the following conditions are met:
- When the deceased is over 80 years of age
- When you have personally cared for the deceased over many months or years
- Where you have observed a gradual decline in his general health and function, with no identifiable disease or injury that contributed to this
- You are certain there is no reason to report the death to the coroner.

The family of the deceased receive a copy of the registered cause of death and this is another reason why the cause of death should be clear and accurate. Bear in mind that an unexpected diagnosis on the death certificate can cause a great deal of distress.

The cause of death must also be written in the medical notes. This is important for subsequent letters to the general practitioner (GP), audit or complaints. Cause of death in the medical notes, death certificate and (if relevant) cremation form must be identical.

Usually, one disease or condition is listed in 1a–c, but several conditions may be listed in 2. If there are more than three diseases in the sequence leading to death, you may write more than one at the end, for example 1c hypertension due to phaeochromocytoma.

Cremation forms

There are three parts to a cremation form. Part A is a request for cremation. Part B is the part junior doctors would normally fill in. It must be filled in by a medical practitioner who cared for the deceased during his last illness and has seen the body after death (by visiting the mortuary if necessary). Part C is completed by an independent doctor who has been registered for at least 5 years. This would be either a GP from a different practice, or a senior hospital doctor not involved in the care of the deceased. The doctor completing Part C must interview the doctor who has completed Part B. Both doctors must see the body after death.

Some of the questions on a cremation form seem difficult for the first time (partly because of the use of obscure words such as 'pecuniary' and 'ordinary' medical attendant). The medical notes are needed to complete a cremation form accurately.

The questions in Part B of a cremation form are:

- *Have you, so far as you are aware, any pecuniary interest in the death of the deceased?* Pecuniary means financial – the answer to this should be 'no'.
- *Were you the ordinary medical attendant of the deceased?* This means 'were you the GP?'
- *What examination of (the body) did you make (after death)?* The answer to this is usually 'external'.
- The cause of death should be listed identically to that on the death certificate.
- *What was the mode of death?* You are then given some examples: syncope, coma, exhaustion, convulsions, etc. The answer to this should be based on your knowledge of the patient and/or reading of the medical notes. Some patients die suddenly (syncope), some slowly fade away, for example, in pneumonia or advanced cancer (exhaustion), some are comatose, for example, in liver failure or large strokes (coma).
- *By whom was the deceased nursed during his or her last illness?* An example answer is 'Ward 1 nursing staff, St Elsewhere's General Infirmary'. However, you must also give at least one name of a member of the nursing staff in this section. You will find this in the 'nursing notes' section of the medical notes, as the event of the death will have been recorded here by the nurse on duty at the time, as well as other names (e.g. lead/primary nurse).
- *In view of the knowledge of the deceased's habits and constitution, do you feel any doubt whatever as to the character of the disease or cause of death?* This question is double-checking that there is no possible neglect, violence, poisoning or other unnatural circumstances related to the death. The answer should be 'no' – otherwise a referral to the coroner is required.
- *Has a pacemaker or any radioactive material been inserted in the deceased? If so, has it been removed?* Unremoved pacemakers cause damaging explosions in crematoria so you must ensure that any have been removed before completing the cremation form. Normally the mortuary staff will remove any pacemakers or radioactive implants if requested.
- Your *registered* qualifications are those held on the General Medical Council database, usually MB ChB (not your BSc and MRCP, etc.).

Key points: Death certification and the coroner

- A death certificate is an important legal and epidemiological document.
- Discuss all causes of death with a senior doctor before completing a death certificate.
- Remember to write the cause of death in the medical notes as well.
- Certain causes of death must be referred to the coroner.
- A cremation form is a legal document and the cause of death should be identical to that on the death certificate.

Exercises

1 Which of the following causes of death require referral to the coroner?
  (a) Community acquired pneumonia
  (b) Pneumonia following a fractured neck of femur
  (c) Death from pneumonia within 24 hours of admission from a nursing home
  (d) Aspiration pneumonia caused by acute alcohol intoxication
  (e) Hospital acquired pneumonia
2 Which of these are unacceptable causes of death on a death certificate?
  (a) Gram negative septicaemia
  (b) Multiple organ failure
  (c) Pneumonia
  (d) End-stage heart failure
  (e) Old age

Answers

1 (b), (c) and (d) require referral to the coroner
2 (a), (b) and (d) are modes of death rather than causes of death

Reference

1. The Home Office. *Reforming the Coroner and Death Certification Service: A position paper*. March 2004. www.homeoffice.gov.uk

CHAPTER 12

Fitness to drive

> **By the end of this chapter you will be able to:**
>
> - Recognise the medical conditions which affect fitness to drive
> - Be able to refer to the DVLA guidelines when advising patients

The guidance described below refers to the current Driver and Vehicle Licensing Agency (DVLA) rules in the UK, which are updated every 6 months. Up-to-date information can be accessed from www.dvla.gov.uk/at_a_glance/content.htm

Audits show that doctors frequently forget to give advice about driving. In the UK, it is the duty of the doctor to advise patients that they have a condition to which the rules apply. It is the duty of the *patient* to inform the DVLA and it decides on each case.

In the interests of road safety, those who suffer from a medical condition likely to cause a sudden disabling event at the wheel or who are unable to safely control their vehicle due to any other cause, should not drive. In some countries, it is up to the doctor as to whether or not a patient is fit to drive. In the UK, fitness to drive is governed by law and this law is interpreted by a medical advisory panel on behalf of the Department of Transport.

Definitions

The Road Traffic Act 1988 refers to prescribed, relevant and prospective disabilities:
- A *prescribed* disability is one that legally prevents a person from holding a driving licence (e.g. recurrent seizures).
- A *relevant* disability is a medical condition likely to render a person a source of danger while driving (e.g. a visual field defect).
- A *prospective* disability is a medical condition which, due to its progressive or intermittent nature may develop into a prescribed or relevant disability in the course of time (e.g. insulin-dependent diabetes). A driver with a prospective disability may normally only hold a driving licence subject to medical review every 1–3 years.

In the UK, a group 1 licence is for motorcars and motorbikes. A group 2 licence includes large lorries and buses. You should always ask what type of driving licence a patient holds, as the rules for group 2 drivers are more strict. An ordinary (group 1) licence is held until the age of 70 years; after that the driver must renew it every 3 years.

When patients do not follow advice about driving

Although it is the duty of the licence holder to notify the DVLA of any medical condition which may affect his safety to drive, sometimes the licence holder cannot or will not do so. In these circumstances, the General Medical Council (GMC) has issued guidelines which allow doctors to breach patient confidentiality in the interests of public safety. This would ordinarily be done by a senior doctor. The following steps are taken:

- First of all, ensure the patient understands he has a condition which may impair his ability to drive. Make sure he knows this is the law and that he is required to inform the DVLA, and you are not just giving medical advice which may be ignored by a competent adult.
- If the patient is incapable of understanding your advice (e.g. because of dementia) you should inform the DVLA yourself.
- If the patient refuses to accept the diagnosis or the effect of the condition on his ability to drive, you can arrange a second opinion, but he should not drive until this has been obtained.
- If the patient continues to drive when he is not fit to do so, even after you have tried to persuade him (including involving his next of kin if the patient allows it), you should inform the DVLA. You should normally inform the patient of your intention to do so, and write to him to confirm it afterwards.

Strictly speaking, a license holder may continue legally to drive until the DVLA has completed its investigation and come to a decision about fitness to drive. But there are certain disabilities (e.g. recurrent blackouts) when it may be *medically* inadvisable to drive during this time. If a patient continues to drive against medical advice, this would invalidate his insurance. So in practice, patients are asked not to drive from the time they are medically assessed and to inform the DVLA as soon as possible.

There are some conditions where they may be 'mitigating circumstances'. For example, a person may have had a provoked seizure due to prescribed medication which he is no longer taking. In these cases, the DVLA will decide each case on an individual basis, and the mitigating circumstances can be outlined in a medical report which the doctor (normally the consultant or general practitioner) will be asked to provide. It is ultimately up to the DVLA, not the doctor, to decide on a person's fitness to drive.

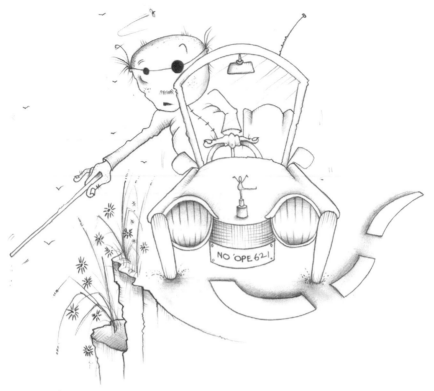

Fitness to drive.

Medical conditions which affect driving

Medical conditions which affect fitness to drive come under the following categories:
- Neurological disorders
- Cardiovascular disorders
- Diabetes mellitus
- Psychiatric disorders
- Drug and alcohol misuse
- Visual disorders
- Respiratory and sleep disorders.

Table 12.1 shows common conditions presenting to the acute take which affect driving. Patients should be asked whether they drive, what type of licence they have, and given the appropriate advice. Note that the diagnosis of some conditions requires a *thorough* history (including from an eyewitness), and the decision to advise a patient not to drive should usually be taken after review by an experienced doctor because many conditions are diagnosed incorrectly (e.g. vasovagal syncope is often confused with seizures). Table 12.1 lists only

Table 12.1 Common conditions presenting to the acute take which affect fitness to drive

Condition	Comments
Seizures	May not drive for 1 year (longer for group 2). 'Seizures' includes all types, for example aura, myoclonic jerks, partial as well as tonic clonic seizures. More than one seizure within a 24-hour period is treated as a single event for the purposes of driving. People who only have seizures during sleep may drive under certain circumstances (see www.dvla.gov.uk).
Provoked seizures	Provoked seizures (apart from caused by alcohol or illicit drug misuse) are dealt with on an individual basis. Provoked seizures include seizures due to medication, eclampsia, reflex anoxic seizures, seizures at the time of head injury or neurosurgery, or at the time of a stroke or TIA.
Coming off epilepsy medication	May not drive for 6 months in most cases.
Transient loss of consciousness	
(a) Obvious vasovagal syncope (except cough syncope)	No restrictions.
(b) Unexplained syncope with low risk of recurrence	This means a thorough history (including from an eyewitness) suggests syncope, and the person has a normal heart and neurological examination. May not drive for 4 weeks (longer for group 2).
(c) Unexplained syncope with high risk of recurrence	Syncope (diagnosed as above) in the presence of heart disease/an abnormal ECG, occurring at the wheel or other 'high-risk factors' (see www.dvla.gov.uk). These people should be investigated by a cardiologist. May not drive for 4 weeks if the cause is found and treated, or 6 months if not (longer for group 2).
(d) Unwitnessed loss of consciousness/altered awareness with 'seizure markers'	Common in the elderly. Markers are defined in the guidance. May not drive for 1 year (longer for group 2).
(e) Loss of consciousness/altered awareness with no clinical pointers whatsoever*	*After evaluation by a specialist. May not drive for 6 months (longer for group 2).
Recurrent disabling vertigo (e.g. Meniere's disease)	May not drive until symptoms are under control.
Stroke (infarct or bleed), TIA	May not drive for 1 month (longer for group 2). Can resume driving without informing DVLA if full neurological recovery after this time. Patients with multiple TIAs must inform DVLA and may not be allowed to drive until symptom free for 3 months.

(*Continued p. 98*)

Table 12.1 (*Continued.*)

Condition	Comments
Asymptomatic benign brain tumours found incidentally	No restrictions for group 1 licence holders.
Neurosurgical procedures, surgery, serious head injuries, intracerebral bleeds, subarachnoid haemorrhages, brain metastases, etc.	Various rules apply (see www.dvla.gov.uk).
Angina at rest or behind the wheel	May not drive until symptoms controlled.
Myocardial infarction	May not drive for 1 month (longer for group 2).
Incapacitating arrhythmia	May drive after 4 weeks if identified and controlled (longer for group 2).
Cardiological procedures and surgery	Various rules apply (see www.dvla.gov.uk).
Disabling hypoglycaemia in diabetes	May not drive until symptoms controlled (insulin users may not hold a group 2 licence).
Acute and chronic psychosis/mania	May not drive until has been well for 3 months (longer for group 2). See www.dvla.gov.uk.
Dementia causing poor short-term memory, concentration and lack of judgement	Decision on driving is based on individual medical reports.
Alcohol misuse and dependency including alcohol-related illness (e.g. cirrhosis)	Defined in the guidance. May not drive until recovery for varying lengths of time (see www.dvla.gov.uk).
Drug misuse and dependency	May not drive until recovery for varying lengths of time (see www.dvla.gov.uk).
Sleep apnoea and cough syncope	May not drive until symptoms controlled.

TIA: transient ischaemia attack.

*This guidance is accurate at the time of writing, but is reviewed every 6 months, and doctors should familiarise themselves with the DVLA website.

common conditions encountered by junior doctors, so you should always be vigilant for any condition that may affect driving and look for the relevant rules regarding fitness to drive on the DVLA website.

Key points: Driving and the DVLA

- All doctors need to be aware of common conditions which affect fitness to drive.
- It is the doctor's duty to tell the patient that his medical condition affects fitness to drive.
- It is the duty of the patient to inform the DVLA.
- In certain circumstances a doctor may breach patient confidentiality in the public interest.

Exercises

- Look at Table 12.1 and discuss whether or not you remember to ask about driving when you see one of these patients.
- Have you ever had to tell a patient that he or she may not drive? What happened?

Self-assessment: Case histories

1 A 70-year-old man is admitted with 'collapse ?cause'. The history is that he had been celebrating his 50th wedding anniversary that day and had an unusually large meal with alcohol. After getting up to go to the toilet in the middle of the night, he collapsed after passing urine. He remembers feeling hot and nauseated, before briefly blacking out. He has a normal heart on history, examination and ECG. What is your advice?

2 A 60-year-old man attends A&E after experiencing left arm weakness and dysphasia for 5 minutes. This is the third time this has happened this week. What is your advice about driving?

3 A 50-year-old alcoholic lady is admitted on the surgical ward with acute pancreatitis. On day 4, she has a seizure. What should she be told about driving?

4 A 50-year-old bus driver is admitted with new onset angina at rest. What should you tell him about driving?

5 A 25-year-old heroin user is admitted because of a groin abscess from repeated injections. He has a full-time job. What, if any, advice about driving is required?

Self-assessment: Discussion

1 This is an obvious vasovagal syncope and does not affect fitness to drive.

2 After a single transient ischaemia attack (TIA) patients may not drive for 1 month. After serial TIAs, patients must stop driving until they are symptom free for 3 months. Serial TIAs are an indication for admission to hospital.

3 Any patient with any type of seizure may not drive. This is likely to be a provoked seizure, due to alcohol withdrawal. If this were a provoked seizure due to medication, the DVLA would assess on an individual basis. However, in the case of alcohol dependence, the patient would not be allowed to drive for a minimum of 1 year.

4 A patient with angina at rest may drive his normal car once symptoms are controlled, but may not drive a group 2 vehicle until he has been symptom free for 6 weeks and met strict exercise test criteria.

5 Heroin users may not drive and have to prove they have been drug free (from any drug) for a minimum of 1 year before regaining their licence. Patients on a properly supervised methadone programme may drive if they are assessed and this is subject to an annual review by the DVLA.

CHAPTER 13

Adult and child protection

> **By the end of this chapter you will be able to:**
>
> • Understand the legal framework relating to adult and child protection
> • Know some of the symptoms and signs of abuse
> • Know about the procedures involved in adult and child protection

Adult and child protection issues are covered in professional guidelines and legislation. General Medical Council (GMC) guidelines state: 'If you believe a patient to be a victim of neglect or physical, sexual or emotional abuse and the patient cannot give or withhold consent to disclosure, you should give information promptly to an appropriate responsible person or statutory agency, where you believe that the disclosure is in the patient's best interests. You should usually inform the patient that you intend to disclose the information before doing so. Such circumstances may arise in relation to children, where concerns about possible abuse need to be shared with other agencies such as social services. Where appropriate you should inform those with parental responsibility about the disclosure' [1].

The Department of Health and the Home Office have issued guidance on adult protection for use by all health and social care organisations, the voluntary sector and police. This states that: 'Abuse is a violation of an individual's human and civil rights by another'. Although any subsequent intervention should take place with the consent of the person being abused (if he or she has capacity), the Department of Health guidance states that 'an individual's wishes cannot undermine an organisation's legal duty to act [2].

Adult protection

Every hospital or primary care trust has a lead clinician in adult protection. Healthcare professionals should discuss any concerns about possible abuse with their senior and members of the multi-disciplinary team in the first instance. These concerns should be handled by an experienced member of staff.

There are several stages in the Adult Protection Procedures:
• A concern is reported by a senior member of staff
• A referral is made to the Adult Protection Enquiry co-ordinator
• A decision is made as to whether adult protection procedures are appropriate

- An enquiry follows
- A plan is agreed as to how the risk of abuse can be reduced
- The plan is reviewed after an agreed time.

If the person experiencing abuse does not have the capacity to make a decision regarding his or her care, an independent advocate is appointed. The Mental Capacity Act 2005 includes statutory powers for the protection of vulnerable adults who do not have the capacity to make decisions on their own behalf. This is discussed in more detail in Chapter 8.

Elder abuse

Elder abuse is thought to be an under recognised and under reported problem. A House of Commons Health Committee report in 2004 indicated that as many as 500,000 older people are being abused in England at any one time [3]. In 2003 a survey of district nurses found that 88% of them had encountered elder abuse in their work [4]. This means that a healthcare professional seeing between 20 and 40 elderly patients a day is likely to see one person who is the subject of abuse of some kind [5].

The following definition of elder abuse has been adopted by the World Health Organisation: a single or repeated act or lack of appropriate action occurring within any relationship where there is an expectation of trust, which causes harm or distress to an older person [6]. This abuse can be in any of the following categories:

- Physical abuse (e.g. hitting, restraining or inappropriate use of medicines)
- Psychological abuse (e.g. threatening or humiliating)
- Financial abuse (e.g. stealing or defrauding someone of goods or money, including benefits)
- Sexual abuse
- Neglect or failing to provide adequate care (e.g. food, heat, hygiene and medical attention).

Most of the above are also criminal offences.

The majority of reports of abuse relate to people living in their own homes, perpetrated by a family member or paid carer (see Box 13.1). Although only 5% of older people live in a care home in the UK, there is a higher than expected number of reports of abuse from institutions.

Box 13.1 Case history

A daughter took on the role of carer for her elderly father. She lived in his house and claimed benefits for looking after him. The patient had been admitted to hospital for a chest infection, and was noted to have lost a lot of weight. No medical cause was found and it emerged that he was being left alone at home without heat, light or food and that he had been physically abused. He was scared of returning home and was moved to a residential home following adult protection procedures.

Recognising symptoms and signs of elder abuse

Detecting symptoms and signs of abuse is difficult, since vulnerable adults are less likely to report abuse and some of the presentations of abuse are common in a frail geriatric population for other reasons. *There are no pathognomonic symptoms or signs of elder abuse.* In addition, abuse may be unintentional. Presentations which may raise suspicions include:
- Disclosure by the patient
- Over use of medication to 'keep the patient quiet'
- Delay in presentation of an injury
- Pattern of injury not consistent with the history given
- Poor personal hygiene and inadequate clothing
- A disparity between the patient's assets and living conditions.

Vulnerable adults are often subject to pressures which influence their right to self-determination. The onset of dementia can affect a person's decision-making abilities. Families may disagree with health professionals or among themselves on the best course of action. Early involvement of a senior doctor, with regular and clear communication is essential in resolving these problems.

Child protection

The British Medical Association (BMA) guidance: 'Doctor's responsibilities in child protection cases' acknowledges that the safeguarding of children not only applies to paediatricians but to all doctors whose work involves children and to those doctors working with adults whose illness or condition may have an impact on the health or well-being of a child [7]. All healthcare professionals have a responsibility to inform a senior colleague should they suspect a child is at risk of harm.

There are two main pieces of legislation relating to the protection of children. These are the Children Act 1989 and the Children Act 2004, shown in Fig. 13.1. Together they make the welfare of a child paramount and the agencies involved have a statutory responsibility to work together for the welfare of children.

Department of Health guidance 'What to do if you are worried a child is being abused' gives clear advice to consult with senior colleagues and refer to social services if concerned [8]. This procedure is outlined in Fig. 13.2.

There has been considerable concern that suspicions which have proved unfounded will put the doctor raising the concern at risk of litigation. A House of Lords appeal judgement dismissed this, stating that the doctor's duty of care is primarily to a child suspected of being harmed and not to the parents. However, the judgement goes on to say, 'The task of the local authority and its servants in dealing with children at risk is extraordinarily delicate ... Social services whilst putting the needs of the child first must respect the rights of the parents; they also must work if possible with the parents for the benefit of the children.... Inevitably a degree of conflict develops between those objectives' [9].

The Children Act 1989	The Children Act 2004
1. The welfare of the child is paramount	'Every Child Matters'
2. Children are best brought up and cared for within their own families	Aimed at transforming children's services and making inter-agency co-operation statutory.
3. Parents with children in need should be helped to bring up their children themselves	Five main aims of the act:
4. Children should be kept safe and protected by effective intervention if in danger	1. Be healthy 2. Stay safe 3. Enjoy and achieve 4. Make a positive contribution 5. Achieve economic well-being
5. Courts should ensure delay is avoided and only make an order where to do so is better than none	
6. Children should be informed about what happens to them	
7. Parents continue to have parental responsibility	

Figure 13.1 Legislation relating to the protection of children.

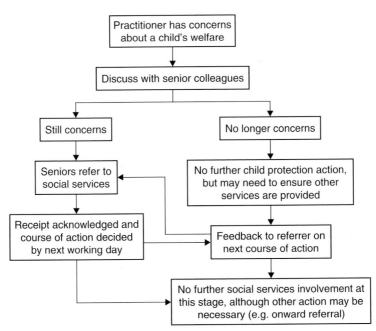

Figure 13.2 Procedures if worried a child is being abused.
Adapted from 'What to do if you are worried a child is being abused – summary' UK Department of Health, 2003.

Recognising symptoms and signs of child abuse

Children are active and frequently have accidents causing injury. They may suffer from a medical condition causing bruising or fractures. On the other hand, some parents do harm their children. *There are no pathognomonic symptoms or signs of child abuse*. Some fractures are highly suggestive but this depends on the history given. Controversy over 'shaken baby syndrome' highlights the point that all injuries could be accidental. Healthcare professionals should be aware of situations which might indicate child abuse, but also be aware that this is a sensitive matter which needs to be handled by experienced professionals. Presentations which may raise suspicions include:

- Disclosure by a child of abuse
- Alleged history of how injury occurred is not developmentally possible
- Delay in presentation of an injury
- Pattern of injury not consistent with the history given
- Poor growth without an organic cause.

In summary, a child's welfare is paramount if there are concerns of abuse. Professionals who work with children have a legal framework and professional guidance on this matter. Always discuss with a senior colleague if you have concerns.

Key points: Adult and child protection

- Healthcare professionals need to be aware that abuse exists and report any concerns to senior colleagues.
- There are legal frameworks and professional guidance on adult and child protection.
- Elder abuse is under recognised and under reported.
- There are certain presentations that raise suspicions of adult and child abuse and require further investigation.

Exercises

- Have you ever come across any situations of possible abuse? What happened?
- Discuss the following case: a 70-year-old man with mild cognitive impairment talked to the occupational therapist. He said that his young neighbour goes to collect his pension every week, does his shopping and takes around 50% of the cash in payment for doing this. Is this abuse?
- Discuss the following case: a 14-year-old girl visiting her grandmother in hospital tells you that she has been sexually abused by her mother's new boyfriend. She then says she does not want you to tell anyone. What should you do?

Self-assessment: Case histories

1 A 2-month-old baby said to have moved from his room on his own to the top of the stairs and fallen down. There is a skull fracture on the X-ray. Is this suspicious?

2 A 8-year-old boy is brought with bruising to accident and emergency by a school support worker. The school support worker wants you to examine him as she thinks he is being abused. What do you do?

3 A frail elderly man with Parkinson's disease is admitted from a nursing home with a chest infection. The ward nurses report that he has extensive pressure sores which were not documented in the nursing home care plan and he appears not to have had any treatment for this. He is malnourished. The particular nursing home has a reputation for poor care. How should you proceed?

4 An elderly lady with severe dementia lives with her husband who has mild dementia. He is her main carer. She is currently a hospital inpatient. In the past he has refused home care on the basis that he can look after her himself. The district nurse is concerned at the state of the house and the patient, who is often found sitting in her own faeces. What can be done?

Self-assessment: Discussion

1 Developmentally, a 2-month old should be socially smiling, fixing gaze and following with his eyes. Children of this age cannot move distances. If placed on the edge of a bed or sofa they may move enough to fall off. This story is suspicious and warrants further investigation by a more senior doctor. However, if the story was that the baby's 5-year-old sister had attempted to carry him down the stairs and accidentally dropped him (which does happen), this is not necessarily suspicious.

2 A person with parental responsibility has legal responsibility for a child (see Chapter 8). If the child has been brought for examination without the parent's knowledge or consent, you cannot examine the child until the parents have been contacted and have agreed to the examination. If they refuse and the school is concerned about abuse, the school must contact social services who will arrange a medical examination with the parents present.

3 The Department of Health has published minimum standards for care homes for older people. If a care home is thought to be neglecting patients by providing substandard care, it can be reported to the local Commission for Social Care Inspection (CSCI) for action [10]. This would be done by a senior member of staff, based on evidence and after discussion with the multi-disciplinary team.

4 Does the patient herself have the capacity to make decisions regarding her own care? If not, is her husband acting in her best interests? If there is evidence of neglect, even unintentionally, a discussion needs to take place

between a senior member of the healthcare team and the husband. Usually, clear communication will result in a plan that keeps everyone happy; for example, the patient can be discharged home as long as the husband agrees to let social services in the house. Are there any other relatives who can help? In extreme cases, the patient can be placed under a Guardianship order and decisions about her care made by local social services.

References

1. General Medical Council. *Confidentiality: Protecting and Providing Information.* General Medical Council, London, 2000.
2. Department of Health. *No Secrets: Guidance on Developing Multi-agency Policies and Procedures to Protect Vulnerable Adults from Abuse.* Department of Health, London, March 2000.
3. House of Commons Health Committee. *Elder Abuse,* London, March 2004.
4. Potter J. *Findings in Relation to the Community and District Nursing Association Survey Examining the Issue of Elder Abuse.* CDNA, London, 2003.
5. Lachs MS and Pillemer K. Elder abuse. *Lancet* 2004; **364**: 1263–1272.
6. World Health Organisation. *The Toronto Declaration on the Global Prevention of Elder Abuse.* World Health Organisation, Geneva, 2002.
7. British Medical Association. *Doctors' Responsibilities in Child Protection Cases.* British Medical Association, London, 2004.
8. Department of Health. *What to Do If You Are Worried a Child Is Being Abused.* Department of Health, London, 2003.
9. House of Lords. *Judgments – JD (FC) (Appellant) v East Berkshire Community Health NHS Trust and Others (Respondents) and Two Other Actions (FC).* House of Lords, London, 2005.
10. Commission for Social Care Inspection. www.csci.org.uk.

CHAPTER 14

Ethical principles in healthcare

By the end of this chapter you will be able to:

- Understand the ethical models used in healthcare
- Use these models to address ethical dilemmas at work

Healthcare professionals are constantly faced with ethical challenges. From the distressed daughter who says, 'Don't tell my mum it's cancer', to the 15-year-old *Jehovah's Witnesses* who refuses a blood transfusion, junior doctors are often the ones patients and their families turn to, as a familiar face readily available on the wards. For a trainee, these ethically and often emotionally charged interactions can seem truly daunting. Senior help is often at hand, but now is the time to start developing your practical skills and flexing those ethical muscles.

Ethics and the law

The law offers a guide to how doctors should act in certain circumstances. But in many situations there may simply be no clear legal precedent. Determining what is the *right* thing to do in your work as a doctor requires something different than an encyclopaedic knowledge of medical law or professional guidelines. Some hospitals have on-call clinical ethicists who provide advice around the clock. However, rather than relying on someone else's judgment, it is important that you have an understanding of the various ethical principles that underpin medical practice and start developing your own ethical framework to tackle these problems in a consistent and reasoned manner.

The Four Principles approach

Probably the best known ethical framework is the Four Principles approach advocated by Tom Beauchamp and James Childress [1]. This gives you a checklist which can help as you weigh up competing ethical demands in any particular situation (see Box 14.1). The principles are:

- Respect for autonomy
- Beneficence (doing good)

> **Box 14.1** Case history
>
> Use the Four Principles approach to work through the following dilemma: an 88-year-old patient with known oesophageal cancer and mild dementia has presented for the second time with haematemesis. She confides in you that she would rather die than have 'another of those horrible camera tests', but her family wants everything to be done and insist that she does not really understand what is happening to her.
>
> **Autonomy**
> Does this patient have the ability to make a fully autonomous decision? You may feel that respecting her right to self-determination is only meaningful if she is unconstrained by her underlying cognitive impairment.
>
> **Beneficence**
> Having the test could help identify the bleeding and stop it. This may help prolong the patient's life, or at least make it more comfortable.
>
> **Non-maleficence**
> The procedure carries risks in itself, and there are 'harms' even if everything goes smoothly (e.g. the unpleasantness of the test). Going against the patient's expressed wishes may be a harm. How significant do you think these factors are?
>
> **Justice**
> Using staffing and facilities to carry out this patient's test may mean others have to wait, which may result in complications for them. What do you consider a fair way of allocating resources in this particular case? Should younger patients have priority?

- Non-maleficence (not doing harm)
- Justice.

The Four Principles approach does not necessarily give an answer, as inevitably there will be competing principles at stake. It merely represents a tool to help you reach a justifiable conclusion in a particular case.

Paternalism

Respect for autonomy (which literally means 'self-rule') is now widely accepted as a pre-eminent ethical principle in healthcare in western societies. There is general agreement that a competent adult has the right to refuse medical treatment, even if it might result in death. However, this is a fairly new development.

Medical paternalism – 'doctor knows best' – had long been the dominant ethic in healthcare and still is today in some countries, with doctors acting in the perceived best interests of patients, often without consultation and even if this goes against the patient's wishes.

Consequentialism

Broadly speaking, this grouping of ethical theories holds that the right action in any situation is one which results in the best balance of good over bad consequences. Although this may seem intuitively appealing as an ethical principle in healthcare, it seems to ignore the inherent 'goodness' or 'badness' of the act itself. For example, giving a patient a lethal injection to put him out of his pain could be justified using the consequentialism approach, irrespective of the motive or nature of the act itself.

Rights-based ethics

Human rights ethics within healthcare have also gained prominence in recent years. The starting point here is a set of absolute or qualified rights which can 'trump' other considerations when deciding how best to act. The Human Rights Act 1998, which incorporated the European Convention on Human Rights in to UK law, has further embedded this approach within healthcare practice.

International declarations

There are a growing number of international statements of principles which are meant to guide doctors in the ethical treatment of patients or research participants. These include the Declaration of Helsinki, which was formulated in 1964 and had its fifth revision in 2000 [2] and the Council of Europe's 1997 Convention on Human Rights and Biomedicine [3].

Key points: Ethical principles in healthcare

- Ethical dilemmas are commonplace in the practice of medicine.
- Law and professional guidelines provide general guidance but cannot assist you in every situation.
- The most commonly used ethical framework is the Four Principles approach: respect for autonomy, beneficence, non-maleficence and justice.
- Ethical dilemmas should always be discussed with a senior doctor.

Exercise

- Describe an ethical dilemma you have faced. Reflect on the outcome and whether using the Four Principles approach would have made a difference.

Self-assessment: Case histories

See how applying the different ethical frameworks described above affects your decision making in the cases described below.

1 An 85-year-old man is admitted with severe pneumonia. He is normally 'fit and well'. The multidisciplinary team is discussing his cardiopulmonary resuscitation (CPR) status. You are asked for your opinion.

2 A 40-year-old man has been in a persistent vegetative state for 7 months following a road traffic accident. His wife wants to talk to you about why he is still being fed by nasogastric tube when she says she knows it is not what he would have wanted. What do you think?

3 A 70-year-old woman is admitted with obstructive jaundice and has a biliary stricture (probably caused by cholangiocarcinoma) stented. Following this she develops biliary peritonitis and several senior doctors decide that she is not fit for surgery. The patient is likely to die within the next few days, but for now is alert and fairly well. Should you tell her that she is dying?

4 You need to move a young patient with severe sepsis from the admissions unit to the high-dependency unit (HDU), but there are no beds. The HDU sister bleeps you to say that she could move one of the elderly, more stable, patients to create a bed, but needs you to okay this first. What issues does this dilemma raise and what do you do?

5 A patient with a stroke which has led to left sided inattention, cognitive and swallowing problems keeps pulling out his nasogastric tube. The nurses mention to you the use of mittens to prevent this. What is your opinion?

Self-assessment: Discussion

1 Using the Four Principles approach, respect for autonomy would require you to ask the patient his wishes, if possible. The conversation should include information on the chances of success of CPR. This is considered good practice and advocated by the UK guidelines on *Decisions Relating to Cardiopulmonary Resuscitation* [4]. However, one might adopt a paternalistic approach and say that the chance of survival to discharge after CPR in such a patient is slim, and any discussion would be upsetting for him, therefore the patient should not be informed of a decision to withhold CPR. Using consequentialism, one might say that it is better to have a quick and painless death towards the end of natural life, than a long drawn out one with disability, therefore the patient should not be for CPR. Then one might consider the Human Rights Act – Article 2 'the right to life', Article 8 'the right to freedom of expression', which includes the right to hold opinions and to receive information vs Article 3 'the right to be free from inhuman or degrading treatment'.

2 Persistent vegetative state is subject to particular guidance. The Courts have identified that referral should be made to them to decide on the lawfulness of withdrawal of nutrition and hydration in persistent vegetative states

rather than being decided by the healthcare team. A number of ethical issues may be raised: the patient's previously expressed wishes, any conflict of interest between family members and the religious beliefs of those involved.

3 Have you ever found yourself avoiding a dying patient, for whatever reason? Nowadays it is considered good practice to be honest and share information with patients. However, in reality doctors tend to talk in coded terms and find it hard to eliminate even a small glimmer of hope. Some patients make it clear that they do *not* want to know and their wishes must be respected. Sometimes, it is relatives who ask you not to tell. Such requests are usually misguided and lead to a conspiracy of silence that causes strain and guilt for all concerned. It should be made clear to relatives that you will not withhold information from the patient unless the patient wishes it. The different ethical frameworks described above may lead to different decisions in this case.

4 The National Service Framework for Older People [5] contains eight standards and the first one is 'rooting out age discrimination'. It states that: 'NHS services will be provided, regardless of age, on the basis of clinical need alone'. However, doctors are continually having to make decisions based on the scarce provision of HDU facilities in the UK. Any patient who is more stable may have to be moved in less than ideal circumstances to make way for another. Use the different ethical approaches to see what decisions you come to in this case.

5 Restraint is sometimes used for adults who lack capacity to make decisions regarding their healthcare under a doctor's duty of care in order to protect the patient's safety or the safety of others. The restraint should be the minimum possible and only used after careful consideration and never out of convenience. Some stroke units have formal policies on the use of mittens and procedures which must be followed, involving senior staff and discussion with relatives. You would need to discuss this with the patient's consultant first. Use the different ethical principles to form an opinion on this issue.

References

1. Tom Beauchamp and James Childress. *Principles of Biomedical Ethics*, 5th edn. Oxford University Press, Oxford, 2001.
2. www.wma.net/e/policy/b3.htm
3. http://conventions.coe.int/treaty/en/treaties/html/164.htm
4. www.bma.org.uk/ap.nsf/Content/cardioresus
5. Department of Health. *National Service Framework for Older People*. Department of Health, London, 2002.

Further resource

- Rai GS (ed.). *Medical Ethics and the Elderly. A Practical Guide*. Harwood Academic Publishers, Amsterdam, 1999.

CHAPTER 15

Advance directives

By the end of this chapter you will be able to:

- Understand the legal position of an advance directive
- Know about the practicalities of an advance directive

Advance directives are decisions made whilst a person has capacity about what care they wish to receive if they later lose the capacity to make decisions about their care. The idea of advance directives is to allow people to retain some autonomy about the medical care they receive.

An advance directive is a legally binding decision that relates to the future care of an individual if they do not want a particular treatment. Section 24 of the Mental Capacity Act further defines an advance directive as 'a decision made by a person ... when he has the capacity to do so, that if at a later time and in such circumstances as he may specify, a specific treatment is proposed ... and at that time he lacks capacity to consent to the carrying out or continuation of that treatment, the specific treatment is not to be carried out or continued' [1].

An advance directive may also relate to an individual's request for future treatment. This is *not* legally binding as in law medical practitioners are not bound to give any treatment that they do not believe is in the patient's best interests, or is unlawful [2]. However, it is good practice to take the advance directive into consideration when deciding on best interests and any appropriate treatment.

A competent patient aware of all the facts can refuse treatment, even if this will result in harm or death [3]. Treatment against a competent patient's wishes is assault.

Luttrell summarised the elements needed for a valid advance directive [4]:

- The person has to be a competent adult when they make the refusal
- The person knew the nature and consequences of the refusal at the time that he made the decision
- He was not acting under undue influence at the time of the decision
- The refusal has not been revoked subsequently
- The person is now mentally incapable of making the decision.

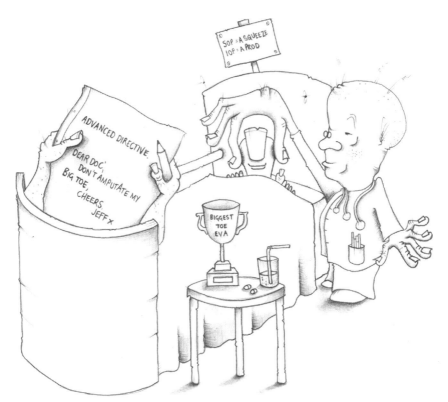

Advance directives.

Box 15.1 Exceptions to advance directives in Case Law

An advance directive does not apply when:
- The person revokes it (this does not need to be done in writing)
- The advance directive does not refer to the specific situation at hand
- During pregnancy where a viable foetus may be harmed as a result
- A doctor does not know that an advanced directive exists.

A doctor will not be liable if he withholds a treatment believing a relevant advance directive exists [5]. The exceptions to advance directives in Case Law are outlined in Box 15.1.

What does an advance directive look like?

An advance directive is normally a typed statement signed by the patient and often witnessed by the general practitioner (GP) or solicitor. A copy is normally held by the GP and a person nominated by the patient to speak on

Box 15.2 A typical advance directive

To whom it may concern
This directive is made by (name) of (address)

I am fully aware that I have (condition) and that it is a progressive condition with no cure. At a time when I am of sound mind and after careful consideration I declare that if at any time the following circumstances exist, namely:
- I am unable to communicate
- I have become unable to participate in decisions about my medical care, and
- Two independent doctors (one a consultant) are of the opinion that I am unlikely to recover from severe illness or impairment involving or expected to cause me severe distress or incapacity for rational existence.

Then and in those circumstances, my directions are as follows:
- That I am not subjected to any medical intervention or treatment aimed at prolonging or sustaining my life
- That any distressing symptoms (including any caused by lack of food and fluid) are to be fully controlled by appropriate palliative care, ordinary nursing care, analgesics or other treatments, even though that treatment may shorten my life, and
- That all directions are to be followed in accordance with my wishes.

I consent to anything proposed to be done or omitted in compliance with the directions expressed above and I absolve my medical attendants from any civil liability arising out of such acts or omissions.

I nominate (name/address) as the person to be consulted by my doctors when considering what my wishes would be in any uncertain situation.

Name and address of GP
Signed
And witnessed by two people, one is usually the patient's GP or solicitor.

his behalf. Organisations such as Dignity in Dying (formerly the Voluntary Euthanasia Society) and the Motor Neurone Disease (MND) Association provide advance directives for people to fill in and advice on advance directives or 'living wills' generally [6].

A typical advance directive is shown in Box 15.2.

Many patients do not have a formal advance directive, but may have told their relatives what they would want in a certain situation. It is always good practice for doctors to talk with close relatives about what a patient would want if he is unable to communicate or lacks the capacity to do so. In many ways, advance directives merely reinforce good communication and help the doctor know that these are truly the patient's wishes.

Clauses 24 to 26 of the Mental Capacity Act clarify the situation around advance directives and ensure that abuse of the process is less likely by introducing safeguards aimed to protect vulnerable people, carers and professionals.

Key points: Advance directives

- An advance refusal of treatment is legally binding.
- An advance request for treatment is not, but should be considered carefully.
- An advance directive is valid if made by a competent adult who is now incapable.
- Advance directives are formal documents, signed by the patient and usually witnessed by a GP or a solicitor.
- If there is any uncertainty about the validity of an advance directive, discuss it with your senior or medical defence organisation.

Exercises

- Have you ever come across an advance directive? What were the circumstances? How did you know that the directive was valid?
- Discuss whether you think a doctor's religious beliefs should affect his judgement when it comes to obeying an advance directive?

Self-assessment: Case histories

1 A 70-year-old man who is unresponsive with a severe stroke once told his wife that if he ever had an incurable condition and was unable to communicate he would not want artificial feeding. He is unlikely to recover any independent function. His children want him to be tube fed and say that you are letting him die from starvation. Would you commence artificial feeding?
2 A 20-year-old lady who is a Jehovah's Witness has come to the Accident and Emergency department after a serious road traffic accident and requires a blood transfusion. In her notes is a formal advance directive stating that she does not want to receive blood products. Would you give her a blood transfusion?
3 A short while later her fiancé arrives, who is a Muslim, and tells you that she was planning to convert to Islam. Would you give her a blood transfusion now?
4 A person is sectioned under the Mental Health Act and has written an advance statement about what treatment he would like to be given. Would you give him the drugs that he has requested?

Self-assessment: Discussion

1 If a person has clearly stated that he does not want a particular treatment then this should be respected. Ideally this should be documented. You

would need to consider whether there is a chance of recovery and the patient's request was intended for this circumstance. This is a difficult situation and there should be a lot of dialogue between senior medical staff and members of the family.

2 No, it would be assault.

3 This was a real case, when a lady who had previously stated she did not want a blood transfusion because she was a Jehovah Witness, became critically ill. She was planning to convert to Islam and thus was going against her previous religion. It was held that her advance decision was therefore void. A person is able to revoke an advance directive in writing or in behaviour at any time. However, you should not assume that things are so simple. People may still hold strong beliefs about blood products whatever their religion. Involve a senior colleague.

4 Any advance statement should be considered when a treatment plan is being made, but doctors are not obliged to provide any treatment at the request of a patient, if it goes against their clinical judgement. However, the British Medical Association (BMA) code of practice points out that such statements should be used in deciding appropriate treatment – this patient may be aware that a particular medication works better for him. An advance directive refusing treatment for a psychiatric disorder does not apply if the person is detained under the Mental Health Act.

References

1. The Mental Capacity Act 2005. www.opsi.gov.uk/acts/en2005/2005en09
2. The Law commission. www.dcagov.uk
3. Re B consent to treatment: Capacity 2002 Child and Family Law Quarterly 14.
4. Luttrell S. Living wills do have legal effect provided certain criteria are met. *British Medical Journal* 1996; **313**: 1148.
5. British Medical Association Guidance (1995/2001): Advance statements about medical treatment – code of practice. www.bma.org.uk
6. www.dignityindying.org.uk, www.livingwill.org.uk and www.mndassociation.org

CHAPTER 16

End of life issues

By the end of this chapter you will be able to:

- Understand the challenge of end of life issues
- Know the law and guidelines in this area
- Understand the issues around 'not for CPR' decisions
- Know how to avoid conflict over care

The challenge

Advances in medicine and rising public expectations have brought about the increasing 'medicalisation' of both life and death [1]. At one extreme, life can be maintained indefinitely without any possibility of reversing underlying pathology or improving quality of life, thereby perpetuating the suffering that medicine was originally intended to address.

The scientific question of how life can be prolonged has been replaced with the ethical question of whether it should, a challenge for even the most experienced doctor. Expanding public knowledge, a shift in the balance of power from medical paternalism to patient rights, and a climate of mistrust triggered by a series of medical scandals all serve to accentuate this challenge. It is inevitable therefore that decision making at the end of life can be complex, is increasingly scrutinised and sometimes contentious.

Pressure to actively maintain life may come from several sources without consideration of the harm of interventions which only briefly delay an inevitable death. Offering false hope, or failing to involve the patient in an informed choice as to how his life should end can also be harmful. How then does a doctor steer a path between these problems, and at the same time deal with uncertainty, and grapple with his own values, prejudices and beliefs?

When considering end of life issues a doctor has to understand:
- Points of law
- Professional guidelines [2,3]
- Ethical principles (autonomy, doing good, not doing harm, justice).

The law and professional guidelines

Guidelines generated by professional bodies are an important point of reference, translating both the law and the ethical principles into a workable format.

The legal case involving a football stadium victim, who was resuscitated to survive in a persistent vegetative state, established the lawfulness of withdrawing artificial nutrition and hydration (ANH) as a means of terminating an individual's life. This resulted in guidelines which gave authority to doctors to either withhold or withdraw ANH in certain circumstances without the authorisation of the courts. However, these guidelines were later challenged by a patient suffering from a progressive neuro-degenerative disorder, who argued that doctors should not hold ultimate authority over such a significant decision. His legal challenge failed, but the legality of the professional guidelines was uncertain for a while.

Double effect

Doctors can care for the dying by giving medicines for pain and agitation which may have the 'double effect' of also hastening death. But any act by one person *intending* to end the life of another is illegal. There is a difference in law between an act of omission (withdrawal of treatment in certain circumstances) and a positive action intended to end life (e.g. injection of potassium chloride).

Euthanasia

Assisted dying for the terminally ill (or euthanasia) is a contentious issue which is currently the subject of much public and Parliamentary debate. The arguments against assisted dying have been viewed as significant enough to override the ethical principle of autonomy. Recent cases of euthanasia in the press have included:

- A patient with advanced motor neurone disease who unsuccessfully sought a ruling from the English and European courts that her husband would not be prosecuted if he helped her take an overdose when she was no longer able to do this unassisted.
- A retired general practitioner suffering from a neuro-degenerative disorder who travelled to Switzerland for an assisted death, where this is legal.

Debate on euthanasia does makes reference to the provision of specialist palliative care services. However, it is argued that for some, a slow death even with good palliative care does not equate with a good death.

Ethics

In end of life decision making, the doctor must first reach a precise diagnosis by considering the patient's:

- Physiological reserve
- Co-morbidities
- Response to treatment
- Treatment options and complications
- Likelihood of success of treatment.

These medical considerations are then combined with the doctor–patient relationship and ethical principles (see Chapter 14). For the competent patient, respect for autonomy is the determining principle, within the law. Only the patient can decide on his quality of life as people vary in their opinion of the tolerability of a disease, medical treatment or disability. The doctor's responsibility in this situation is to present jargon-free information and allow the patient and his family time to reach a conclusion. However, respect for autonomy does not mean that the doctor behaves like a waiter, simply offering options. Patients and their relatives need guidance as well – for example, if a patient is dying and referral to intensive care is inappropriate, this should be clearly stated.

Best interests

When a patient lacks capacity to make decisions himself, unless a relevant advance directive has been made, the ethical principles of beneficence (doing good) and non-maleficence (not doing harm) become more important than autonomy. This equates to 'best interests', discussed in Chapter 8 in detail. The role of the next of kin in these circumstances is complex. Current law gives them no authority but professional guidelines require the involvement of the next of kin, since 'best interests' extends beyond medical best interests and should accommodate the values and beliefs held by the patient whilst competent. Although they cannot determine treatment, the immediate family are usually able to give the most informed view on the patient's values and quality of life when treatment options are being debated.

It is important to explain that a patient is not going to be simply abandoned by the medical team if a decision is made to limit treatment. If the time comes when a patient has deteriorated despite treatment, the *goals* of treatment change from curative to palliative. There should be no hesitation in addressing the needs of a patient with symptoms such as pain. Every medical specialty has the support of a local palliative care team, and hospitals have specialists in pain management.

Not for cardiopulmonary resuscitation decisions

The British Medical Association, Resuscitation Council (UK) and Royal College of Nursing guidelines on decisions relating to cardiopulmonary resuscitation (CPR) open with the words: 'CPR can be attempted on any person whose cardiac or respiratory functions cease. Failure of these functions is part of dying and thus CPR can theoretically be attempted on every individual prior to death. But because for every person there comes a time when death is inevitable, it is essential to identify patients for whom cardiopulmonary arrest represents a terminal event in their illness and in whom attempted CPR is inappropriate. It is also essential to identify those patients who do not want CPR to be attempted and who competently refuse it' [3].

Unrealistic expectations

Many people get their knowledge of CPR from television, which has far better outcomes than reality and tends to portray CPR as a successful 'treatment' [4]. Outcome following in-hospital cardiac arrest depends very much on the condition of the patient. Most cardiac arrests in hospital occur in the context of a serious multi-system illness. Non-shockable rhythms are more likely and these have a very poor prognosis. Sometimes people confuse withholding CPR with withholding all treatment and it needs to be explained that any decision about CPR is totally separate from decisions about other treatment [5].

Pre-empting decisions

Discussing end of life issues with patients long before any life-threatening deterioration respects their autonomy, clarifies their opinion and values and benefits the next of kin, who do not have to second-guess what the patient would want if he cannot speak for himself.

Doctors and relatives would be helped further if patients were able to express their views on other end of life issues such as:

- Organ donation
- Post-mortem examinations
- Retention of tissue and organs for research
- Whether they wish to be cremated, buried or donated to the medical school.

It is uncertain whether society is ready to accept such specific questions but if the ultimate goal is to promote patient autonomy and eliminate uncertainty and substituted judgement, then these changes in the doctor–patient relationship have to be debated.

In chronic progressive diseases such as chronic obstructive pulmonary disease or degenerative neurological conditions, respect for autonomy means informing the patient of the prognosis long before any life-threatening complications occur. This allows the patient to prepare himself for eventual death, forces the explicit consideration of quality of life issues, and clarifies the patient's perspective on the benefits vs harm of any interventions.

In geriatrics, questions about CPR have been proposed as part of the routine clerk-in, as part of an 'ethical' history which also includes questions about religion and which relatives the patient is happy for the doctor to talk to. Many older patients have already thought about death before coming to hospital.

Conflict over care

Conflict over care can arise at the end of life. When a patient does not have the capacity to make his own decisions, the doctor has to balance accommodating the family's perspective with being the ultimate decision maker with the rest of the healthcare team. Communication can be complicated by internal family disagreements, religious beliefs or negative past experiences. Sometimes family members can have unrealistic hopes of recovery.

When any conflict arises, the most important thing is to initiate regular, high-quality communication. Senior doctors should be involved at an early stage. Communication involves listening to the family's perspective, eliciting concerns and offering a consensus medical opinion on the disease, prognosis, treatment options and recommended course of action. An absolute position or a fixed time frame for decisions should be avoided, since this can be interpreted as a play for power and control, and trigger an equal and opposite reaction. Likewise, a declaration that the patient will follow a fixed pattern of deterioration over a fixed time may prove incorrect and trigger mistrust.

Good communication

Communication should start with an explanation of the patient's condition, progress or otherwise, treatment options and likely prognosis, and only when the next of kin have understood and accepted this information should the discussion move to end of life issues.

The term 'futility' should be used with caution as family members may take this to mean that the patient's life is not worth saving. In the first instance, it would be reasonable to suggest that in the event of progressive deterioration despite appropriate treatment, CPR would be inappropriate and to explain why. If the family can accept this, it would then be reasonable to talk about limitations of treatment, perhaps at a subsequent meeting. It is important to emphasise that the patient would continue to receive all other care and treatment to relieve pain and distress. Most families, if given sufficient time, communication and support, will ultimately ask for the patient to be kept comfortable rather than being kept alive by invasive interventions when death is inevitable.

Rarely a consensus cannot be reached. Seeking a legal endorsement of the preferred medical approach will only serve to polarise opinions further, but may be necessary as a last resort. Other options include giving the family time to understand and accept the situation and mediation.

One of the major avoidable sources of conflict is inappropriately optimistic information given to patients and their relatives. On the intensive care unit in particular, doctors from other specialties may not have the experience to give an accurate picture of what the treatment options and prognosis are. It is vital that doctors from different teams communicate with each other before speaking with relatives so that the information conveyed is accurate and consistent.

Key points: End of life issues

- Decision making at the end of life can be complex.
- Doctors need to understand the law, professional guidelines and ethical principles when considering end of life issues.
- When a patient is dying, treatment goals change from curative to palliative.
- Any deliberate act to end life is illegal.
- If a patient is competent, his autonomy should be respected.
- If a patient is not competent, his best interests should be considered in consultation with the family and multi-disciplinary team.
- CPR is not a treatment for death.
- Patients diagnosed with a progressive disease should have the opportunity discuss end of life issues well in advance.
- Conflict over care does arise and can be avoided by good communication.

Exercises

- The Assisted Dying Bill proposes that patients who are terminally ill can request euthanasia. What do you think about this?
- Describe a situation you have encountered where there was disagreement among the clinical team, or between the team and the patient or relatives about an end of life issue.
- What is your experience of communication (by yourself or others) in end of life issues?

References

1. Illich I. *Limits to Medicine. Medical Nemesis: the Expropriation of Health*. Marion Boyars, London, 1976.
2. General Medical Council. Withdrawing and Withholding Life-Prolonging Treatment. Good Practice in Decision Making. General Medical Council, London, 2002.
3. A joint statement from the British Medical Association, the Resuscitation Council (UK) and the Royal College of Nursing on decisions relating to cardiopulmonary resuscitation. www.bma.org.uk/ap.nsf/Content/cardioresus
4. Diem SJ, Lantos JD and Tulsky JA. Cardiopulmonary resuscitation on television. Miracles and misinformation. *New England Journal of Medicine* 1996; **334**: 1578–1582.
5. www.bma.org.uk/ap.nsf/Content/cprleaflet

CHAPTER 17
NHS complaints procedure

By the end of this chapter you will be able to:

• Understand the NHS complaints system

The National Health Service (NHS) (complaints) Regulations 2004 sets out the legal framework for dealing with complaints in the NHS. Each NHS Trust or practice should have arrangements for dealing with complaints. The arrangements are intended to be 'open, fair, flexible and conciliatory and should encourage communication on all sides' [1].

Who's who in the complaints system

The NHS complaints system is designed to investigate complaints with the aim of satisfying complainants and improving systems, rather than apportioning blame.

The following people can make a complaint:
• The patient
• A person who is affected or likely to be affected by an action, omission or decision of the Trust or practice which is subject to the complaint
• A person acting behalf of another (with permission if that person has capacity).

A person complaining on behalf of another without his consent (because the patient lacks capacity or is deceased) must have sufficient interest in the patient's welfare or must be a person with parental responsibility in the case of a child.

Each NHS Trust has a member of the board of directors with responsibility for ensuring compliance with the complaints procedures, a complaints manager, very often a Patient Advice and Liaison Service or PALS (see Box 17.1) and of course, front-line staff such as general practitioners (GPs), consultants and ward managers.

The Department of Health guidance on the NHS complaints system states that, 'At all times NHS staff should treat patients, carers and visitors politely and with respect. However, violence, racial or sexual harassment should not be tolerated. Neither will NHS staff be expected to tolerate language that is of a personal, abusive or threatening nature' [1].

> **Box 17.1** Patient Advice and Liaison Service (PALS)
>
> - PALS is like the 'citizens advice bureau' for the NHS
> - It is an independent and confidential service for patients, families and carers
> - It offers advice, information and support
> - It deals with complaints, suggestions or queries
> - It liaises with other departments to help address problems quickly.

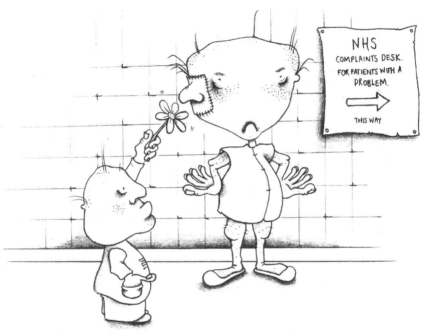

NHS complaints procedure.

The complaints procedure ends if a complainant instigates formal legal action. The matter is then handed over to the NHS body's solicitors.

What happens once a complaint is made?

A complaint can be made verbally or in writing. It may be made to front-line staff, the general practice manager, PALS, the Matron or complaints manager. Very often, complaints can be resolved by front-line staff to the satisfaction of the complainant. However, many people feel uncomfortable making complaints directly to the people involved, and prefer to speak to PALS or write a letter. Very often, the complainant is merely raising areas of concern rather than wishing to make a formal complaint. All formal complaints must be acknowledged in writing within 2 days.

Complaints must be made within 6 months of the event, or within 6 months of the matter coming to the attention of the complainant. If a complaint is made outside this time, the complaints manager may choose not to investigate it, in which case the complainant can ask the Healthcare Commission to consider it. Each complaint is taken on its own merit and a response is given accordingly.

If a complaint is not immediately resolved by front-line staff, the complaints manager may investigate by finding out what took place and keep a file on the matter. A conciliatory meeting may be arranged, for example, between the complainant and the consultant or GP involved, if this is felt to be helpful. A written response is prepared by the complaints manager and this should be shared with the healthcare professionals involved or named in the complaint.

If the complainant is not satisfied with the response, he can ask the Healthcare Commission to review the complaint. Alternatively, the Healthcare Ombudsman can be contacted. The Ombudsman is independent of the NHS and the government. People should normally have complained directly to the NHS body before complaining to the Ombudsman, but the Ombudsman can take complaints directly in exceptional circumstances.

Key points: NHS complaints procedure

- The complaints system is designed to satisfy complainants and improve systems.
- Every NHS Trust has a complaints manager.
- A competent patient's consent is needed if someone else complains on his behalf.
- Very often, complaints are made to raise areas of concern.
- A written response prepared by the complaints manager should be shared with the healthcare professionals involved.

Exercises

- Discuss your experience of complaints in the NHS. What happened? Could the matter have been dealt with differently?
- Describe how you like to be treated when you have a complaint (for example in a shop or restaurant).

Self-assessment: Case histories

1 A relative comes to the desk on the ward to complain that her mother's spectacles have been lost. They were new and cost £150. What is your reply?
2 The ward sister receives a letter to say how horrified a relative was at the standard of care on the ward. His elderly mother appeared neglected, having to wait before her soiled sheets were changed, food was put in front of her

and then removed uneaten half an hour later, and it seemed difficult to get information – he was fobbed off with 'the doctors will be round later if you would like to talk to them'. How should the ward sister respond?

3 A relative comes to the desk on the ward and starts to complain that his wife is in pain. He appears to be intoxicated with alcohol and makes personal and threatening remarks. How should you respond?

4 A patient complains that her diagnosis was delayed and as a result suffered irreversible harm. The letter is addressed to the chief executive and the patient states her intention to sue the hospital for damages. How should the complaint be handled?

Self-assessment: Discussion

1 Put yourself in the relative's shoes. Apologise and say you will get someone who can deal with the matter.

2 Have you ever been a hospital visitor? Sometimes the standard of care is not as it should be. Wards appear chaotic and messy. Things which concern visitors may not be noticed by the staff. There is an 'expectation gap' in terms of information – visitors expect to be given information, whereas staff expect visitors to come and ask for it. This complaint raises lots of issues about the ward system and methods of communication from which the ward sister can learn and change.

3 Always try to diffuse a potentially violent situation by remaining calm and non-threatening. However, this behaviour is unacceptable. If necessary get help, tell the visitor that his behaviour is unacceptable and call security to escort him off the premises. Then go and see the patient by herself.

4 Once a complainant instigates legal action, the NHS complaints procedure does not apply. The letter will be acknowledged and handed over to solicitors. However, this letter only says the patient intends to sue and could be an attempt to get an explanation and an apology for what happened. This could be explored further.

Reference

1. Department of Health. *Guidance to Support Implementation of the National Health Service (Complaints) Regulations 2004.* www.dh.gov.uk

PART III

Clinical Governance and Patient Safety

CHAPTER 18

Why things go wrong

By the end of this chapter you will be able to:

- Understand the frequency of adverse events in healthcare
- Understand the nature of medical error
- Appreciate the importance of incident reporting
- Know the definition of clinical governance

Patient safety is an important issue, yet until recently there has been little research on this subject in the UK. Other industries (e.g. aviation, nuclear power) have learned a great deal about the nature of error and their experience is helping healthcare organisations learn about patient safety.

The scale of the problem

Because of the under reporting of patient safety incidents, there is no clear estimate of the number or nature of errors that occur. A pilot study in a London hospital estimated that 10% of inpatient episodes led to an adverse event [1]. An adverse event was defined as an unintended injury caused by medical management rather than the disease process itself. Around half of the adverse events were deemed preventable. In most cases the patient was minimally affected, but in 8% of cases the adverse event contributed to death. Each adverse event led to an average of nine additional days in hospital, with a cost of nearly £300,000.

Apart from extrapolating from this small study, what else do we know about error in healthcare? The Harvard Medical Practice Study in the USA found that 3.7% of hospital admissions led to adverse events [2,3]. The Quality in Australian Healthcare Study found that 16.6% of admissions experienced adverse events, half of which were considered preventable [4]. In the UK, data also exists from confidential enquiries, complaints, the Medical Devices Agency and the Medicines Control Agency (via the yellow card reporting system at the back of the British National Formulary – BNF) [5]. These data show that:

- There were 6600 adverse events, including 432 serious injuries or death, involving medical devices in 1999

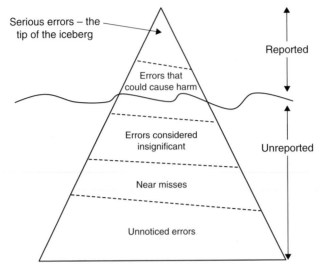

Figure 18.1 The adverse event iceberg.

- 10,000 patients experience a serious adverse drug reaction each year
- There are 20,000 perioperative deaths each year
- There were 38,000 complaints about primary care and 28,000 complaints about secondary care in 1998/1999
- The National Health Service (NHS) paid £400 million in clinical negligence settlements in 1998/1999.

Currently, we can only *estimate* the frequency and nature of adverse events in the NHS. But studies suggest that in the UK there are at least 850,000 adverse events each year and that half of these are preventable.

However, the frequency of medical error (as opposed to adverse events) is far higher. This is because errors may go unnoticed, or be intercepted. Errors are less likely to be reported when the patient has not come to any harm. It has been estimated in industry that there is 1 major injury and 29 minor injuries for every 300 'no harm' accidents [6]. The importance of this is that experience in the aviation industry shows that we can learn far more from these near misses than from the smaller number of serious adverse events that occur. Fig. 18.1 shows the adverse event iceberg that exists in the NHS today. Box 18.1 includes some definitions.

Even if a 600 bed hospital managed to eliminate drug prescribing errors by 99.9%, it would still experience 4000 drug errors a year [7]. Error is inevitable in a complex system such as healthcare. Systems that do not adjust for this can end up exacerbating rather than limiting error. Research also shows that it is not the error rate itself, but measures to rectify errors that are important. Organisations which take steps to look for and rectify errors when they do happen can reduce the consequences of those errors [8].

> **Box 18.1** Definitions
>
> A serious untoward event is an incident involving NHS staff, patients or visitors which results in serious consequences. These must be reported and investigated. Examples include:
> - A death (including suicide) or serious injury
> - The absconsion of a patient detained under the Mental Health Act where there is a risk to the patient or others
> - An incident which is part of a pattern of reduced standards of care
> - An incident which results in serious damage to property or disruption of services
> - Serious fraud.
>
> A critical incident is any other incident which results in harm, for example, an assault, adverse drug reaction, equipment fault. A near miss is an incident which does not result in harm, for example, wrong patient sent to theatre but intercepted in time.

Error chains

Notice so far that we have been talking about 'error' rather than 'mistakes'. This is because research shows that there is usually no *single* cause which explains an adverse event. Instead, errors occur as a result of:
- Faulty systems
- Faulty equipment or technology design
- Lack of resources
- Poor information or communication
- Inappropriate delegation
- Fatigue
- Staff being unaware of safety policies.

The death of a young boy from an accidental injection of intrathecal vincristine has been well documented and is an example of how a series of errors led up to the final adverse event [5]. Other well-known examples of 'error chains' include the Herald of Free Enterprise ferry disaster (a car ferry capsized outside the Belgian port of Zeebrugge with the loss of 188 lives in 1987), the Kegworth air crash (a Boeing 737 crashed on to the M1 in 1989) and the Ladbroke Grove train crash (a passenger train passed a red signal and collided with a high-speed passenger train just outside London in 1999).

A 'red flag' is a term which means 'warning' or 'alert'. We talk about red flags when we talk about error chains. Red flags which are typically found in error chains include:
- Ambiguity
- Poor/conflicting information or communication
- Confusion
- Departure from standard procedure

- Fixation or preoccupation
- Unease
- Denial or irritability
- Inaction
- Equipment alarms.

Sometimes events proceed so quickly, there is little time to prevent an adverse event. But research from aviation shows this is often not the case. With the use of black boxes in aircraft, researchers were able to analyse the response of the crew in the 20 minutes or so before a crash. These red flags were typically present.

A popular model of adverse events is the 'Swiss Cheese' model [5]. This shows all the defences which can protect against an adverse event. These defences can have holes in them – service delivery problems or care delivery problems. When the holes happen to align, an error chain can turn into an adverse event. This is illustrated in Fig. 18.2.

Some of these holes are 'active', for example ignoring a safety policy, but many are 'latent' – conditions that are always present and can be difficult to correct. Examples of latent failures relevant to doctors in training are:

- Design of on-call rotas (e.g. the on-call specialist registrar (SpR) has to be in two places at once)
- Inadequate or incorrect equipment
- Staff shortages
- Poor information systems or poorly maintained medical records
- Inadequate training (e.g. practical procedures)
- High turnover of staff
- Fatigue [9]
- The practice of handling unlabelled syringes

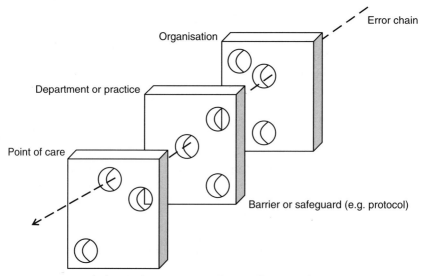

Figure 18.2 How 'holes' in the system can align to allow an adverse event.

- Lack of communication protocols
- The hierarchical nature of acute medical care (e.g. the first port of call for an acutely ill patient is the most junior doctor).

Because of a lack of understanding regarding adverse events, the NHS has concentrated on people as a cause of error. So an adverse event was followed by disciplinary action, more training or the introduction of rigid guidelines. Sometimes, this may be appropriate, but this approach fails to look at the root causes of error. 'To err is human' is the name of an important report published by the Institute of Medicine in the USA on this subject [10]. Errors are inevitable even in the best organisations. They also tend to recur in patterns. Therefore, we need to consider a more effective way of tackling error, which concentrates on the latent failures which are present, things which may even seem normal because they have been there for so long. 'Root cause analysis' is the name given to the method of analysing adverse events in this way.

In root cause analysis, a small team is assembled to ask the questions 'what, how and why?' of a patient safety incident. The aim is to get to the fundamental

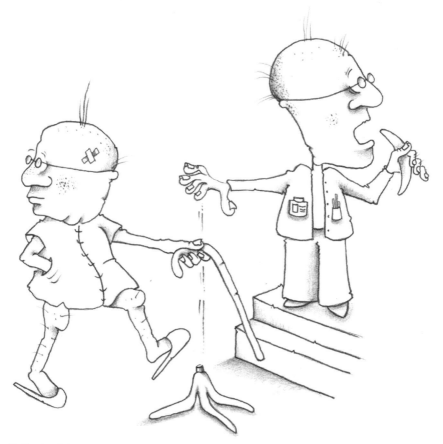

Patient safety.

root of the problem in order to prevent similar incidents from happening again. Serious incidents, frequently occurring incidents or near misses are appropriate for root cause analysis. The first task of the group is to gather information from people, policies and procedures, medical records and other sources. The group can then use a number of methods to gain consensus on the organisational, context/departmental and human factors which surrounded the incident. Causal and influencing factors are identified. Following this, the group makes recommendations aimed at strengthening systems (safeguards), preventing errors (holes) and reducing the impact of adverse incidents if they do happen.

Reporting incidents

The only way to prevent medical error is to know about the frequency, nature and root causes of error. To be able to do this, the NHS needs an effective incident reporting system that not only reports serious adverse events, but near misses as well. The latter are 'free lessons' on the nature and causes of error. An effective reporting system [5] should be:
- Entirely separate from any disciplinary or regulatory body
- Easy to use
- Standardised within an organisation
- Confidential
- Mandatory
- Part of a culture where individuals are thanked for reporting incidents.

Currently, less than half of NHS Trusts provide training on risk management or reporting and less than a third provide guidance to staff on what to report [11]. As a consequence, the rates of incident reporting vary widely.

You may already be familiar with your Trust's incident reporting system. For example, these are the forms that nursing staff fill in after a patient has fallen in hospital and injured himself. Critical incidents and near misses are also reported using these forms. Serious untoward events have a separate system. Under reporting is widespread, so many doctors feel uncomfortable in reporting incidents or feel as if they are blaming someone instead of helping to improve the system. Regular feedback may not occur and staff doubt whether reporting makes any difference.

Below are some broad categories in which incident reporting would be appropriate (but there are many more):
- Prescribing errors
- Adverse drug reactions
- Equipment faults or problems with availability
- Injury as a result of a practical procedure
- Near misses (e.g. wrong patient arrives in theatre)
- Absent medical records
- Patient care affected for non-clinical reasons
- Assault
- Needlestick injury.

The National Patient Safety Agency

The National Patient Safety Agency (NPSA) was set up in 2001 to co-ordinate the efforts of the entire NHS to report, and more importantly learn from, error and problems which affect patient safety [12]. The role of the NPSA is to:

- Collect and analyse information on adverse events from local NHS organisations, staff, patients and carers
- Assimilate other safety related information (e.g. from confidential enquiries and other reporting systems)
- Learn lessons and ensure these are fed back in to practice
- Produce solutions to prevent adverse events, specify national goals and monitor progress.

The NPSA promotes patient safety, incident reporting and an open learning culture. It has its own on-line incident reporting system which NHS staff can use [13], as well as collecting data from Trusts. It also promotes education and research in patient safety and offers training in root cause analysis with courses or on-line modules [14].

Clinical governance

The term 'clinical governance' refers to the means by which an entire organisation ensures it delivers high-quality care. Prior to 1997, chief executives of healthcare trusts were legally responsible for financial governance but not clinical governance (standards) in their organisations. New legislation, national clinical standards and monitoring systems were introduced to ensure that clinical governance would be implemented [15]. Fig. 18.3 shows the current clinical governance structure in the NHS.

Clinical governance has several components. From a junior doctor's perspective, audit, induction, protocols and training programmes are the most visible part of clinical governance. For a consultant or general practitioner (GP), national guidelines, standards, inspections, appraisal and revalidation are also important. Each Trust has a designated clinical governance lead.

The clinical negligence scheme for Trusts (CNST) was established to provide a means for NHS Trusts to fund the cost of clinical negligence litigation. Membership is voluntary and it is open to all NHS Trusts in England. Members pay into a central fund, but get a discount if they can show that they meet the CNST's clinical risk management standards. There is a greater discount for Trusts that meet higher standards.

The standards are in the following categories:
- Learning from experience (adverse events, complaints and national reports)
- Response to major clinical incidents
- Advice and consent
- Medical records
- Induction, training and competence
- Clinical care
- Mental health services.

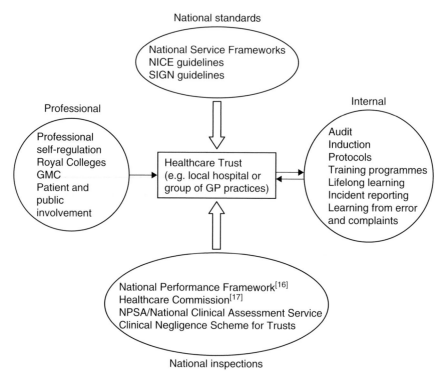

Figure 18.3 Clinical governance structure in the NHS. GMC: general medical council; NICE: National Institute for Clinical Excellence; SIGN: Scottish intercollegiate guideline network.

Trusts are inspected and scored using a detailed list of standards in each of these categories which cover systems and protocols, staff training and assessment (including junior doctors), incident reporting, infection control and medicines management.

Poorly performing doctors

Although most adverse events occur as a result of faulty systems, it is estimated that around 5% of doctors perform below the standards defined by the profession [16]. Clinical governance systems do not necessarily pick up poorly performing doctors. Identifying doctors whose knowledge, skills and attitudes are below standard can be difficult but can result from:
- Complaints from patients and colleagues
- Litigation
- Performance that significantly departs from 'normal' medical practice
- Audit (e.g. high level of post-operative complications)
- 360° appraisal.

There are a number of reasons why a doctor may perform poorly [17]. These include:

- Physical illness
- Stress, depression and other mental illness
- Drug and alcohol dependency
- Workload, including sleep loss
- Lack of necessary education and training
- Poor practice management, infrastructure or resources
- Poor relationships with colleagues
- Attitudinal problems.

Normally, it is a pattern, rather than a single incident, which raises doubts about a doctor's performance. It is vitally important that steps are taken to help the doctor concerned and to protect patients as soon as possible. For doctors in training this involves initially the educational supervisor, then the Foundation Programme director or Deanery, or the General Medical Council (GMC) for serious problems or criminal offences. For consultants and GPs this involves initially the medical director and NHS employer, then the National Clinical Assessment Service (NCAS) which offers an objective assessment, advice, support and mediation or the GMC. The GMC has the power to remove a doctor's name from the medical register.

Key points: Why things go wrong

- Adverse events are common.
- An adverse event is more likely to be due to a chain of errors rather than a mistake by one individual.
- Errors are more likely when there are latent failures in the system with inadequate safeguards.
- Red flags can alert you to the fact that you might be in an error chain.
- Even if the NHS was nearly perfect there would still be adverse events, so minimising the impact of adverse events when they do occur is also important.
- Clinical incident reporting is an important part of clinical governance.
- The NHS has a clinical governance structure.
- Most errors are made by good doctors; a minority of doctors perform poorly and should be dealt with as soon as possible.

Exercises

- Think of some 'latent holes' which are present in the system where you work – these are ways of doing things which may even seem normal because they have always been done that way, but could easily lead to an adverse event in the right circumstances (see previous list for examples).
- Describe an adverse event which you have been involved in. In retrospect, what could have prevented this (a) in the system (b) at the point of care? Was an incident form filled in?

- Perform a mock 'root cause analysis' with some colleagues. Choose an adverse event of which you have some knowledge.
- Look at the list of latent failures relevant to doctors in training. Can you identify with this? What could be done differently to prevent these?
- Have you ever found yourself in the middle of a potential error chain but not fully realised at the time? Look at the list of red flags and describe any incidents that come to mind.

References

1. Vincent C, Neale G and Woloshynowych M. Adverse events in British hospitals: preliminary retrospective record review. *British Medical Journal* 2001; **322**: 517–519.
2. Brennan TA, Leape LL, Laird NM, Hebert L, Localio AR, Lawthers AG *et al.* Incidence of adverse events and negligence in hospitalised patients. *New England Journal of Medicine* 1991; **324**: 370–376.
3. Leape LL, Brennan TA, Laird NM, Lawthers AG, Localio AR, Barnes BA *et al.* Incidence of adverse events and negligence on hospitalised patients: results of the Harvard medical practice study ll. *New England Journal of Medicine* 1991; **324**: 377–384.
4. Wilson RM, Runciman WB, Gibberd RW, Harrison BT, Newby L and Hamilton JD. The quality in Australian healthcare study. *Medical Journal of Australia* 1995; **163**: 458–471.
5. Department of Health. *An Organisation with a Memory. Report of An Expert Group on Learning from Adverse Events in the NHS.* Department of Health, London, 2000. www.dh.gov.uk
6. Heinreich HW, Peterson D and Roos N. *Industrial Accident Prevention*, 5th edn. McGraw-Hill, New York, 1980.
7. Leape L. The preventability of medical injury. In: Bogner MS (ed.). *Human Error in Medicine*. Lawrence Erlbaum Associates Inc, New Jersey, 1994.
8. Silber J, Rosenbaum P, Schwartz J, Ross R and Williams S. Evaluation of the complication rate as a measure of care in coronary artery bypass surgery. *Journal of American Medical Association* 1995; **274**: 317–323.
9. Association of Anaesthetists of Great Britain and Ireland. Fatigue and Anaesthetists. www.aagbi.org/guidelines.html
10. National Academy of Sciences. Linda R, Janet C and Molla D (eds). *To Err Is Human: Building a Safer Health System*. National Academy Press, Washington, DC, 2000.
11. Dineen M and Walsh K. *Incident Reporting in the NHS. Health Care Risk Report*. 1999; **5**(4): 20–22.
12. www.npsa.nhs.uk
13. www.npsa.nhs.uk/health/reporting
14. www.npsa.nhs.uk/health/resources/root_cause_analysis
15. Department of Health White Paper. *The New NHS. Modern. Dependable*. Department of Health, London, 1997.
16. Donaldson LJ. Doctors with problems in an NHS workforce. *British Medical Journal* 1994; **308**: 1257–1258.
17. Cox J, King J, Hutchinson A and McAvoy P (eds). *Understanding Doctors' Performance*. Radcliffe Publishing, Oxford, 2006.

CHAPTER 19

Human factors

By the end of this chapter you will be able to:

- Understand the term 'human factors'
- Understand how the performance of teams relates to patient safety
- Know how lessons from the aviation industry are applicable to healthcare

'Human factors' is an umbrella term used to describe the way people interact with each other, their systems and technology. The basic concepts of human factors were originally researched and designed by the aviation industry and are immediately applicable to healthcare [1], as the stories throughout this chapter illustrate (see Box 19.1).

Research in military and civil aviation shows that human factors play a significant role in the majority of accidents. Accident analyses, simulator research and cockpit voice recordings show that unsafe flight conditions are frequently related to failures in cognitive and social skills rather than lack of technical knowledge. One analysis of 119 fatal air accidents revealed the following causes (more than one in many cases) [2]:

- Inadequate communication – 41%
- Deviating from standard operating procedures – 37%
- Maintenance deficiency – 15%

Box 19.1 Everyday human factors

A 20-year-old lady with severe asthma and several previous intensive care unit admissions was about to be transferred from Accident and Emergency (A&E) to the admissions unit. The doctor decided to accompany the patient. The patient was on 15 l of oxygen via a non-rebreathe bag. The porter arrived with a chair and an oxygen cylinder but the doctor noticed that the oxygen cylinder dial was in the red zone indicating almost empty. The doctor asked the porter to fetch a full oxygen cylinder for the transfer. A disagreement ensued. The porter felt that the oxygen supply would be enough for the transfer. What issues does this story raise?

- No ground proximity warning system – 12%
- Design faults – 11%
- Inadequate training – 11%
- Weather information – 9%
- Others – 24%.

Human factors encompasses the understanding of patterns and causes of error (outlined in Chapter 18), situation awareness, systems, communication within teams and the limitations of human performance.

Situation awareness

For example, a light aircraft is heading towards an airport surrounded by mountains. The captain has inadvertently descended below the minimum safe altitude and the aircraft is on a collision course with the mountain. It is the co-pilot's first day and he can see that the aircraft is heading for the mountain. The captain is experienced and has flown this route many times before. He is bored and pre-occupied with problems at home. The co-pilot reasons that such an experienced captain surely knows what he is doing. Is there any need to say anything?

Situation awareness involves knowing what is going on around you and being alert to potential problems. Individuals have situation awareness, just like the co-pilot, but groups also need situation awareness. Often a team's situation awareness can be low because no one communicates. Situation awareness is compromised by:

- Poor/conflicting information or communication
- Confusion (e.g. over roles and responsibilities)
- Departure from standard procedures
- Distractions
- Inexperience
- Poor training
- Poor interpersonal skills/attitude
- Physical and emotional fatigue and stress.

Systems

Systems are important too. Patient safety is more likely to be put at risk because of a combination of faulty systems, equipment, resource problems, fatigue and poor training which all combine to form an error chain rather than one member of the healthcare team making a mistake. Faulty systems increase the likelihood of error, whereas safety conscious systems provide safeguards against error (see Box 19.2). When safeguards are weak, latent holes appear, as described in the previous chapter.

Communication within teams

Communication within teams is important (see Box 19.3) and one aspect of this has been discussed in Chapter 5. In terms of human factors, communication includes:

- Confirming roles and responsibilities
- Anticipating the needs of others

Box 19.2 The Harvard Monitoring Standards

In the late 1970s anaesthetists used a stethoscope to ensure that a patient was being effectively ventilated. But a series of deaths caused a risk management committee to be formed which looked at all the events that occurred over a 10-year period. It found that the vast majority of preventable adverse incidents due to anaesthesia were due to a failure of ventilation. In 1985 the Harvard Monitoring Standards were introduced which made it mandatory to continuously monitor ventilation. The use of end-tidal carbon dioxide measurements (capnography) was strongly encouraged and became mandatory in the USA in 1995. This simple standard has reduced deaths due to anaesthesia and is an example of how systems can be strengthened in order to improve patient safety [3].

Box 19.3 Clearly articulating safety concerns

During a night shift in one large hospital there are six doctors covering general medicine: two house officers, three senior house officers (SHOs) and one specialist registrar (SpR). The workload is divided between the admissions unit, respiratory medicine and care of the elderly. The care of the elderly SHO is overwhelmed by admissions, some of whom are seriously ill. The other two SHOs have no one waiting to be seen and the SpR is reviewing non-urgent cases. The care of the elderly SHO needs help, but does not call anyone. What points does this story illustrate?
- Clearly articulating safety concerns
- Culture (not wanting to call for help)
- The effects of fatigue on performance
- Leadership (or lack of it).

- Co-operating
- Verbalising concerns
- Communicating plans
- Giving clear instructions
- Calling for help if needed
- Listening to others
- Resolving conflict in a non-confrontational manner.

The limitations of human performance

Human factors also involves an understanding of the limitations of human performance. With the advent of 'hospital at night', the Association of Anaesthetists of Great Britain and Ireland [4] and the Royal College of Physicians of London [5] have produced guidelines on fatigue for night workers. However, workload,

---

Box 19.4 Tunnel vision?

A 50-year-old man was having a laparoscopic repair of an umbilical hernia under general anaesthesia. While the surgeon was placing the trocar in the abdomen, the patient suffered a cardiac arrest (pulseless electrical activity). Whilst cardiopulmonary resuscitation (CPR) was carried out, the team went through the possible causes of the patient's deterioration. The surgeon was sure that he had not entered the peritoneum and therefore could not have damaged an intra-abdominal blood vessel, so air embolus was considered the most likely cause (a recognised complication of this procedure). Five minutes later another member of staff arrived who had come across a similar incident previously, due to a damaged intra-abdominal blood vessel. He asked the surgeon to open up the abdomen. A discussion ensued about whether to do this. The member of staff insisted. They found a lacerated iliac artery which was repaired and the patient made a full recovery.

---

stress and ill health also affect performance and doctors need to recognise this and ask for help if needed.

In simulated scenarios and real life incidents it is apparent that a tunnel vision can sometimes develop which prevents effective decision making, communication and team performance. For example, a person may be absolutely sure that he executed a procedure correctly and therefore not consider all possibilities or accept suggestions (see Box 19.4).

What is normal?

Healthcare staff get used to cutting corners and executing procedures in an unacceptable and unsafe manner because it has always been done that way. They were trained that way, they are short staffed, the right equipment is often not available and unsafe practice becomes 'normal'. Because there is a general low team situation awareness and a culture which does not pay attention to near misses, these latent failures are an accident waiting to happen (see Box 19.5). Chapter 18 described 'active' and 'latent' holes in systems which allow errors to slip through barriers or safeguards.

For example, a common latent failure is the inadequate observation of vital signs in hospitals. Healthcare students are not taught how to measure and interpret vital signs to a standard required for patient safety. Vital signs are an important measure of how ill a person is. Many vital signs are measured (or not) by healthcare assistants. Until recently, there were no systems which enabled inexperienced staff to recognise seriously abnormal vital signs and oblige them to call for help [6]. An article which graphically illustrates this latent failure is listed in Further resource at the end of this chapter.

Box 19.5 'Normal' practice

An otherwise fit 80-year-old man was admitted with chest pain to the local admissions unit. The SHO who clerked him in made a diagnosis of an acute coronary syndrome. As part of the ethical history, the SHO had asked about CPR and the patient indicated that he would like to have CPR if the need arose. The SHO assessed that the patient was high risk on the basis of age and electrocardiogram abnormalities so thought about where the patient should be observed.

The SHO explored the options. The cardiac monitors available on the ward were old and often did not work. The alarms were always switched off because they kept sounding due to movement artefact. The ward was short staffed and most of the nurses were unsure how to read a cardiac monitor. The SHO indicated that the patient should be moved to a bed opposite the nurses' station, but this never happened because the staff were busy and forgot and the SHO finished his shift at 5 p.m. and did not hand over. The SHO had considered whether to refer the patient to the cardiology department, but reasoned that the department only had one coronary care unit bed which was being saved for someone who might need to be thrombolysed. Moving the patient to cardiology would necessitate an ambulance ride to another wing of the hospital, plus the patient was 80 years old which (the SHO thought) made it less likely that he would be accepted. The SHO in the end reasoned that the patient would probably be okay on the admissions unit.

The patient stayed where he was and had an unwitnessed cardiac arrest during the night and died.

There are several points raised in this story to do with systems and human factors, but one of the most important is this: because a practice seems normal does not mean it is acceptable or safe. In this story, problems included:
- Longstanding problems with equipment
- Inadequate training for an admissions unit
- Inadequate staffing for an admissions unit
- No doctor-to-doctor handover at 5 p.m.
- No referral to cardiology because of the anticipation of rejection
- Procedures which allowed patients with chest pain to be admitted to an area remote from cardiology
- Not enough speciality beds for workload
- Ageism, whether perceived or real
- No clear articulation of safety concerns
- Relying on luck rather than safe practice.

Human factors awareness and training can help us all distinguish normal from unsafe practice and to articulate safety concerns on behalf of patients.

Team resource management

Training programmes called 'crew resource management' have been introduced in the aviation industry, designed to increase the use of non-technical skills and improve safety. Flight crews work on a shift pattern with different people, rather like hospital staff. They need good non-technical skills (as well as technical skills) in order to work effectively together. The most similar medical speciality to aviation is anaesthesia because of the use of checklists, simulation in training and a set of skills which is in many ways similar to flying an aircraft. In theatre, up to 80% of critical incidents are related to human factors rather than lack of technical knowledge or equipment failure. Research in anaesthetists' non-technical skills (ANTS) is ongoing [7], but teaching and assessing ANTS involves team training in the classroom and during simulated scenarios. Analysis of ANTS shows that non-technical skills fall in to four domains:

1 Task management
2 Teamwork
3 Situation awareness
4 Decision making.

For example, under the heading of teamwork is the ability to co-ordinate activities with other team members. This includes confirming roles and responsibilities and communicating clearly with other members of the team. It is easy to make assumptions about getting things done or to intervene without informing others, practices which can easily lead to error (see Box 19.6).

However, all clinical teams need 'crew resource management'. The advantages of such training become particularly apparent in an emergency. Think of the last cardiac arrest or trauma call you attended. Research in this area shows that good leadership and communication are particularly important if the situation is not to degenerate in to a confusing free-for-all. Whilst each member

---

Box 19.6 Too many chefs
A novice anaesthetist was assisting the consultant during an emergency laparotomy. The operation had started and the patient's blood pressure was low because of severe sepsis. A noradrenaline infusion was started to treat hypotension. The consultant decided to give a small bolus of noradrenaline because of profound hypotension. Just after he had done so, the novice, who had not seen him give the bolus, had the same idea. The consultant saw the novice finish giving the bolus and it was then that they realised what had happened. A moment later the patient developed severe hypertension and tachycardia, causing ST depression on the electrocardiogram.

of the team may be technically competent, the entire team has to work together to be safe, effective and efficient. One of the concepts taught to pilots in training is: always establish who is flying the aircraft.

Essentially, crew resource management is a set of countermeasures to protect against human error [8]. For example, if this were implemented in the National Health Service, all front line staff would receive regular training in issues related to human factors and safety issues, including the use of simulations where task management, teamwork, situation awareness and decision making are assessed. Team members would be trained to communicate in ways which maximise safety and minimise the possibility of misinterpretation, assumption, different mindsets or errors. For example:

- A team briefing takes place before each shift where the team leader outlines the plan, any anticipated problems, roles and responsibilities
- Staff are trained to always verbalise safety concerns
- Staff are trained to listen and respond appropriately to safety concerns
- Staff monitor each other's behaviour by double checking (e.g. drawing up and labelling intravenous drugs)
- Instructions are verified by repeating them aloud.

Simple elements such as briefings which establish a shared mental model, an emphasis on safety, cross checking and communication protocols form part of a bigger picture which is a shared understanding of the nature of error, human factors, leadership and teamwork. These non-technical skills are as important in delivering effective care as medical knowledge, especially in high stress, high stakes emergency situations.

Key points: Human factors

- Human factors refers to the way people interact with each other, their systems and technology.
- Human factors play a significant role in adverse events.
- Human factors training involves: the patterns and causes of error, situation awareness, systems, communication within teams, the limitations of human performance and prioritising safety.

Exercises

- You are part of the hospital at night team. Think of the differences and advantages in adopting a crew resource management system for 1 week of nights.
- A senior colleague is demonstrating a practical skill without a proper sterile technique. How could you address this in a non-confrontational manner?
- Look at the causes of the air accidents at the beginning of the chapter. Can you think of any medical situations in which these causes resulted in a critical incident or a near miss?

- Discuss ways of promoting teamwork in your workplace.
- Describe a situation that you have been in where your or another's situation awareness was compromised by the factors described in the list above.

References

1. Global Air Training. www.globalairtraining.com/health.htm
2. McAllister B. *Crew Resource Management. Awareness, Cockpit Efficiency and Safety*. Airlife Publishing Ltd, Shrewsbury, 1997.
3. Eichhorn JH, Cooper JB, Cullen DJ, Maier WR, Philip JH and Seeman RG. Standards for patient monitoring during anaesthesia at Harvard Medical School. *Journal of the American Medical Association* 1986; **256**: 1017–1020.
4. The Association of Anaesthetists of Great Britain and Ireland. Fatigue and Anaesthetists 2004. www.aagbi.org/guidelines.html
5. Horrocks N and Pounder R. *Working the Night Shift: Preparation, Survival and Recovery*. The Royal College of Physicians of London 2006. www.rcplondon.ac.uk/pubs/books/nightshift
6. Cooper N, Forrest K and Cramp P. Patients at risk. *Essential Guide to Acute Care*, 2nd edn. Blackwells, Oxford, 2006.
7. ANTS website www.abdn.ac.uk/iprc/ants.shtml
8. Musson and Helmreich. Team training and resource management. *Harvard Health Policy Review* 2004; **5(1)**: 25–35.

Further resource

- An article by a consultant anaesthetist who experienced being seriously ill as an in-patient. Sanai L. As others treat me. *BMJ Career Focus* 2006; **332**: 68–69.

CHAPTER 20

Safe prescribing

> **By the end of this chapter you will be able to:**
> - Follow the simple rules for safe prescribing
> - Know common drug error situations
> - Understand the concept of concordance

Many patients have problems which are related to their drug treatment, for example dizziness, renal impairment or dyspepsia. In the elderly population iatrogenic conditions are extremely common. Therefore, as a doctor you should never just prescribe a patient's usual medicines without thinking about each drug and whether it should be prescribed at all, or at the same dose (see Box 20.1).

In 1996, a study in general practice found that 66% of repeat prescriptions were not authorised by a doctor and 72% had not been reviewed in the previous 15 months [1]. Patients should have their prescriptions reviewed on a regular basis.

One of the fundamental roles of a doctor is to prescribe. Being unable to prescribe safely and have a working knowledge of pharmacology is like being a blind surgeon. The Foundation Programme syllabus outlines the basic competencies that all new doctors are expected to demonstrate when it comes to prescribing, and these are shown in Box 20.2.

Box 20.1 Writing up usual medicines

A 70-year-old man with hypertension is admitted with sepsis due to ascending cholangitis. On examination his blood pressure is 90/60 mmHg and his creatinine comes back as 200 μmol/l (previously 90 μmol/l). His usual medicines are: lisinopril 20 mg daily, bendrofluazide 2.5 mg daily, doxazosin 4 mg daily and prn ibuprofen for arthritis pain. How would you write up his usual medicine chart?

In this case, it should be obvious that all his usual medicines should be stopped (as well as the fact that the patient requires resuscitation).

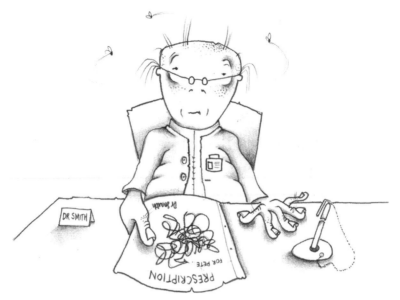

Prescribing.

Box 20.2 Foundation Programme syllabus for safe prescribing

The Foundation trainee should know:
- The effects of patient factors on prescribing (e.g. the elderly, children, pregnant women)
- How to prescribe in renal impairment
- How to prescribe in hepatic impairment
- Common drug interactions
- Common drug error situations
- Drugs which require therapeutic monitoring
- How to prescribe oxygen*
- How to prescribe blood products
- The evidence-base for certain prescribing
- The principles of safe prescribing.

The Foundation trainee should be able to:
- Take an accurate drug history (including allergies) from the patient and other sources
- Work with the ward or community pharmacist
- Use the British National Formulary (BNF)
- Prescribe clearly with a legible signature
- Explain drug therapy to a patient
- Explain common side effects.

*See 'oxygen therapy' in our companion book *Essential Guide to Acute Care*, 2nd edn.

Here are the simple rules for safe prescribing:

- Always write prescriptions in printed capital letters, if you do not use a computerised system
- Use generic not brand names (except for epilepsy medicines)
- Always make a note of allergies – these should be clearly written on the chart
- Always think about interactions before you prescribe
- Make your signature a readable version of your name rather than a squiggle
- Write microgram as 'mcg' and units as 'units'
- Make decimal points clear. 'Trailing' zeros should never be used (e.g. 1.0 mg), but 'leading' zeros should always be used (e.g. 0.1 mg)
- When changing the dose or route of a drug, re-write (do not amend) the prescription
- Prescribe essential drugs via another route if the patient is 'nil by mouth'
- Always check calculations with someone else
- Never write up a drug if you do not know what it is – you are responsible for what you prescribe. Look it up in the British National Formulary (BNF) first
- Fluids are also a drug – check electrolytes before prescribing these.

In your experience, how often do doctors follow these rules?

Common drug error situations

Medication errors are preventable and can occur in the prescribing, dispensing or administration of medicines. They account for up to 20% of all adverse events and cost at least £200 million per year in UK hospitals alone. Drug errors are not the same as adverse drug reactions (e.g. allergies), which may be unpredictable and therefore unavoidable. However, there is an overlap, as illustrated in Fig. 20.1. Box 20.3 lists the common sources of drug error.

Most medication errors do not result in harm. Those that do are the tip of the iceberg, since errors that do not result in harm are unlikely to be reported.

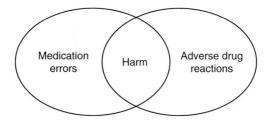

Medication error (e.g. near miss or wrong dose prescribed)
Adverse drug reaction (e.g. allergic reaction or side effect)
Harm (e.g. prescribing a NSAID* to a patient with asthma resulting in an asthma attack, or a different preparation of an anti-epileptic drug by accident, resulting in seizures)

*NSAID: non-steroidal anti-inflammatory drug.

Figure 20.1 Medication errors, harm and adverse drug reactions.

Box 20.3 Common sources of drug error

- Writing methotrexate once a day (it is normally once a week)
- Prescribing drugs that interact with warfarin without adequate monitoring
- Administering medicines using unlabelled syringes
- Administering chemotherapy without proper training
- Prescribing a penicillin without realising (e.g. augmentin, magnapen, tazocin etc) to a patient who is allergic
- Incorrect calculations of drug doses
- Not communicating clearly to the patient and general practitioner (GP) when medicines are changed.

Prescribing a penicillin without realising to a patient who is allergic is a common and serious drug error. Patients should be asked about allergies before prescribing and healthcare professionals need to be aware that there are several antibiotics which contain penicillin.

Systems can be strengthened to make medication errors less likely, and to minimise harm when they do occur. For example:

- Electronic prescribing
- The clear labelling by manufacturers of drugs containing penicillin
- Infusion pumps with alarms
- Having ready-made bags of fluid containing potassium chloride
- Designing containers which do not look alike
- Availability of antagonists (e.g. naloxone).

One study published in the Lancet identified potentially serious prescribing errors in a UK teaching hospital [2]. The doctors who did the prescribing were interviewed in order to analyse the causes of the errors. Most errors were made because of slips in attention, or because prescribers did not apply the rules of safe prescribing. Doctors identified work environment, whether or not they were prescribing for their own patient, poor communication within the team, their own physical and mental well-being and lack of knowledge as risk factors for prescribing errors. However, organisational factors were also identified: inadequate training, a hierarchical medical team, a lack of awareness of prescribing errors and *the low perceived importance of prescribing*. The ways in which an organisation can make prescribing safer are listed in Box 20.4.

Although most medication errors occur at the prescribing stage, dispensing and administration errors also occur. It is estimated that the error rate for oral drug administration in UK hospitals is around 5% of doses [3]. Sources of administration errors include:

- Ambiguous or poorly written prescriptions which are not queried
- Drugs given at the wrong time
- Drugs given via the wrong route (e.g. epidurally instead of intravenously)
- A similar sounding drug is given instead (e.g. hydralazine instead of hydroxyzine)

Box 20.4 Ways of making prescribing safer

- Teach safe prescribing in medical school (e.g. drug names, doses, calculations, routes and interactions)
- Preserve and protect the monitoring role of the pharmacist
- Ensure that the rules of safe prescribing are followed by everyone
- Emphasise the importance of prescribing and transcribing medicines
- Teach common sources of drug error
- Use the consultant ward round or the teaching consultation to reflect on prescribing decisions and build up an experience base in prescribing.

Adverse drug reactions, even well-known ones, should be reported using the Yellow Card System in the back of the BNF to the Committee on the Safety of Medicines. Drug errors should be reported using local or national incident reporting systems.

Box 20.5 Taking an allergy history

When asking patients about drug allergies, always clarify what they mean by 'allergic'. Many patients describe side effects or are able to give only sketchy information which might be really important. For example, an anaesthetist went to assess a patient pre-operatively to find he was wearing an allergy band which said 'anaesthetics'. You need more information than this!

- The wrong preparation is given (e.g. Tegretol instead of Tegretol Retard)
- The wrong infusion rate is calculated
- A drug is not immediately available therefore is not given at all
- Incorrect inhaler technique by the patient.

When medicines are dispensed from the patient's own locker rather than a traditional trolley, administration errors are reduced and this is now commonplace in UK hospitals [4].

As a doctor you should never assume that what you have prescribed is being administered correctly, or taken by the patient at home. It is common in hospital practice to find an abbreviation inserted instead of a signature and this can be easily overlooked. For example (abbreviations may vary in different institutions):

- D – drug not available
- O – omitted
- N – nil by mouth
- R – refused.

In many hospitals, pharmacists check prescriptions and this has been shown to reduce prescribing error. However, as a doctor, you should never rely on the fact that someone else may check your prescriptions for you. It is *your* responsibility to prescribe safely (Box 20.5).

Concordance

Prescribed medication is the most common form of medical treatment, but non-compliance with prescribed medication is a big problem. Despite the potential benefits of medicines, people often do not take them as prescribed [5]. The major factors affecting compliance are:

- Whether the medicine is for prevention or treatment
- How complex the medication regimen is
- Whether there are unpleasant side effects
- Patients' views on their illness and treatment
- Cognitive or physical impairment which affect medicine taking.

Involving patients in managing their own condition is an important aid to compliance. Whereas compliance refers to the patient taking his medicines, concordance refers to the 'whole package' – appropriate prescribing, communication, education and compliance.

Doctors often prescribe medication with only a limited discussion with the patient. The patient will go home, open his medication packet and read a long list of possible side effects in the information leaflet provided. These side effects are not given any context and the reason why the drug was prescribed in the first place may not be clear. Patients are not informed about whether they can vary their medicines according to their lifestyle, or whether it is crucial to take the drug at a certain time each day.

Compliance is improved when patients:

- Understand their diagnosis and treatment
- Agree with the treatment
- Have had queries and concerns explored and addressed.

The Medicines Partnership [6] is a project supported by the Department of Health, set up with the aims that health professionals will view prescribing as something they do jointly with patients and that services and resources will be made available to help patients through education, information and support.

Key points: Safe prescribing

- Prescribing is a high-risk activity.
- All prescribers should have adequate knowledge and skills.
- All prescribers should follow the rules for safe prescribing.
- Prescribers are accountable for what they prescribe.
- Prescribers should understand the frequency and nature of medication error.
- Medication error should be reported using local or national incident reporting systems.
- Compliance with medicines is a big problem and should be addressed using a package of measures, known as concordance.

Exercises

- Have you ever completed a course of antibiotics?
- Whenever you see a patient with a problem, ask yourself whether it could be a side effect of his medication.
- Make a note of every single medication error you come across during the course of a normal working day. How many and what kind of errors were there?
- Inspect drug charts carefully during one ward round and see how many times drugs have not been given because they were not available, the patient was 'nil by mouth', it was omitted or the patient refused it.
- Do the same with fluid prescriptions and see how many are given at the correct rate and on time.
- Reflect on how you communicate with patients when you prescribe a new drug or stop an old one.

References

1. Zermansky AG. Who controls repeats? *Br J Gen Pract* 1996; **46**: 643–647.
2. Dean B, Schachter M, Vincent C and Barber N. Causes of prescribing errors in hospital inpatients: a prospective study. *Lancet* 2002; **359**: 1373–1378.
3. Barber N and Dean B. The incidence of medication errors and ways to reduce them. *Clin Risk* 1998; **4**: 103–106.
4. Department of Health. *Building a Safer NHS for Patients. Improving Medication Safety. A Report by the Chief Pharmaceutical Officer.* Department of Health, 2004. www.dh.gov.uk
5. McGavock H, Britten N and Weinman J. *A review of the literature on drug adherence.* Royal Pharmaceutical Society of Great Britain, London, 1996.
6. www.medicines-partnership.org

Further resource

- Reid JL, Rubin P and Whiting B. *Lecture Notes on Clinical Pharmacology*, 6th edn. Blackwell, Oxford, 2001.

CHAPTER 21

Infection control

By the end of this chapter you will be able to:

- Understand the importance of infection control
- Behave and dress in a way that helps infection control
- Understand about alert organisms and alert conditions
- Prescribe antibiotics responsibly

Infectious diseases are a high priority in the National Health Service (NHS) today. This is due to the rising incidence of healthcare-associated infection (HCAI), the proliferation of antibiotic resistance, the outbreak of diseases such as severe acute respiratory syndrome (SARS) and the possibility of an impending influenza pandemic. This chapter will focus on infection control in terms of HCAIs in hospital. The National Institute of Clinical Excellence (NICE) has produced guidelines on the prevention of HCAIs in the community [1].

Healthcare-associated infections

Nearly 10% of hospital inpatients will suffer an HCAI [1]. These are infections acquired as a result of contact with the healthcare system whether in the community, care homes or hospital. The impact of HCAIs includes increased length of hospital stay, increased morbidity and mortality and a substantial cost – £1 billion per year in England alone. It is estimated that around 30% of HCAIs are preventable.

Why are HCAIs on the rise?
- More people in hospital are seriously ill
- More people with immunosuppression or neutropenia
- Greater use of catheters and lines which breach natural defences
- Higher bed occupancy and movement of patients
- Too few single rooms
- Poor compliance with hand washing
- Reduced standards of ward cleanliness
- Inappropriate antibiotic use in medicine and agriculture.

The commonest sites of HCAI are the [2]:
- Urinary tract 23% (80% of these due to urinary catheters)
- Lungs 22% (most commonly among ventilated patients)

Box 21.1 'Lazy' urinary catheters

A 70-year-old lady is admitted with a serious chest infection. She is unable to mobilise and is incontinent. She has a urinary catheter inserted by A&E staff. As the patient improves, the urinary catheter is forgotten. Seven days later she becomes unwell again with a Gram negative bacteraemia and requires intravenous antibiotics.

Urinary catheters are commonly inserted when a patient is acutely ill but remain *in situ* to conveniently deal with incontinence or because staff forget about them. Catheters should always be removed at the first opportunity. Incontinence is a treatable condition. Patients can be referred to a continence adviser, urologist or geriatrician.

- Wounds 9% (especially if prolonged, complex surgery in a frail patient)
- Blood 6% (60% of these due to intravenous lines)
- Skin 10%.

The current NHS strategies to control HCAIs include the establishment of:
- Good surveillance systems
- Reduced use of urinary catheters, peripheral cannulae and central lines (see Box 21.1)
- Restricted movement and isolation of infected patients
- Strict antibiotic prescribing policies
- High standards of hygiene
- HCAI a key feature of quality inspections.

Infection control

Every hospital has an infection control team (ICT) consisting of doctors, usually microbiologists, and specialist nurses. The ICT is responsible for setting standards, writing policies, surveillance, liaison with public health doctors and audit – but every healthcare worker has the responsibility of ensuring his own practice is safe. Doctors have a bad reputation for infection control measures. It is up to you to correct this! Box 21.2 outlines the standard (or universal) precautions that all healthcare professional should use.

Trying to control HCAI is not new. In the 1800s Semmelweiss demonstrated that doctors delivering babies could reduce the rate of maternal post-partum infection by washing their hands first. Even in today's modern medical world, good hand hygiene alone can lead to a significant reduction in infection rates.

However, audits of hand hygiene show that healthcare staff do not wash their hands before and after touching patients. The reasons for this are due to both systems and individuals:
- Inadequate facilities
- Lack of time
- Poor knowledge of guidelines

Box 21.2

Standard precautions (also called universal precautions)
- Wash hands or use alcohol gel before and after patient contact
- Hand washing with soap and water is essential if hands are visibly contaminated or in the case of spore forming infections such as *C. difficile*
- Use disposable single use gloves if body fluid contact likely
- Use disposable aprons if clothing might come into contact with a patient
- You still need to wash your hands even if you wear gloves
- Dispose of sharps safely.

Hand hygiene
- In addition to the above, remove all wrist and hand jewellery before hand washing
- Cuts and abrasions must be covered with a waterproof dressing
- Fingernails should be short, clean and polish free
- Effective hand washing has three stages: preparation (wetting hands under tepid water before applying soap), washing and rinsing (rubbing vigorously for a minimum of 10 seconds, paying attention to the tips of fingers, thumbs and areas between fingers before rinsing) and drying (with paper towels)
- If alcohol gel is being used instead, the same measures as for the washing stage apply
- Emollient hand cream can be used to protect the skin from the drying effects of regular hand washing.

- Lack of education
- Lack of enforcement.

Scrupulous hand hygiene is the mainstay of infection control. You need to have a mind-set that every patient is a mass of bacteria and you must avoid carrying these to other vulnerable patients. Healthcare workers who develop diarrhoea and/or vomiting must leave work and not return until they have been symptom free for 48 hours.

It is important to remember that the two strongest risk factors linked to HCAIs are the degree of underlying illness (e.g. immunosuppression) and the use of medical devices (e.g. catheters, tubes, central lines). Therefore, a strict aseptic technique is extremely important when you are performing invasive tests or procedures. If you are performing a procedure such as urinary catheterisation or a lumbar puncture in a ward or A&E department, imagine you are in an operating theatre and use the same sterile technique as you would there. It is not acceptable to perform a procedure without the proper sterile technique just because other people do not do so, or the correct equipment (e.g. sterile gowns and towels) are not available [3].

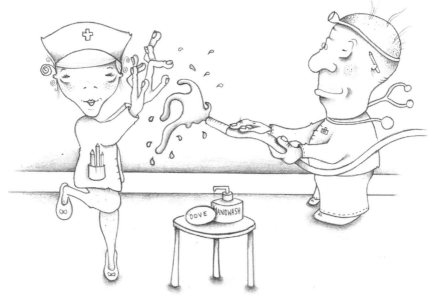

Infection control.

Box 21.3 What to wear at work

The NHS infection control measures require that staff dress appropriately:
- One plain wedding ring (no rings with stones)
- Small stud earrings only
- Short sleeves are preferred
- White coats and ties are a source of debate (they are infrequently washed and trail organisms around) [4].

Correct sharps disposal is very important to reduce the risk of needlestick injuries. Take the disposal bin to the patient and dispose of the sharps there rather than carry them about in search of the ward sharps bin. Ask the ward sister to provide small portable bins if these are not available.

Alert organisms and alert conditions

Alert organisms and alert conditions (e.g. methicillin-resistant *Staphylococcus aureus* (MRSA) and gastroenteritis) may give rise to outbreaks and cause serious morbidity or mortality in susceptible patients (see Box 21.4). You will be warned by the ICT about patients infected with alert organisms. If you suspect

Box 21.4 Alert organisms and alert conditions

Example alert organisms	*Example alert conditions*
• MRSA • Multi-resistant Gram negative rods • Bacterial and viral causes of diarrhoea • Glycopeptide-resistant enterococci • Penicillin-resistant *Streptococcus pneumoniae* • *Mycobacterium tuberculosis* • Group A streptococcus • *Corynebacterium diphtheriae* • Legionella species	• Suspected infective diarrhoea and/or vomiting • Soft tissue infection (e.g. cellulitis) • Tuberculosis • Chicken pox/shingles • Scabies • Fever related to foreign travel and rare infections • Infection with alert organisms diagnosed outside the Trust • Transfers from hospitals abroad (where antibiotic resistance is more common)

an infection with an alert organism, you must ensure the ICT is notified. The affected patients are likely to require a side room and *special* precautions:
• Use of gloves and aprons by all staff
• Adjustment of antibiotic therapy
• Measures to protect other patients
• Explanation for the patient and visitors.
It is also a legal requirement to notify the Centre for Communicable Disease Control (CCDC) about certain diseases which have public health implications (e.g. meningococcal meningitis). Box 21.5 contains the list of notifiable diseases in the UK. The CCDC is usually notified using a form, but meningococcal meningitis is one example where a disease should be notified as soon as possible, for example by telephone.

Specimens and request forms should be labelled with 'infection risk' stickers for patients who might have a blood borne virus infection or other pathogens which can put staff at risk, as outlined in Box 21.6.

Methicillin-resistant *S. aureus*
MRSA is one of the multi-resistant bacteria (often called 'superbugs' in the media). Infection rates vary widely among different hospitals and countries. The Netherlands has managed to almost eradicate MRSA through a policy of 'search and destroy' [5].

The bacterium *S. aureus* has always been a cause of HCAI (e.g. wound infections). However, there is an increasing incidence of *S. aureus* which is resistant to commonly used antibiotics such as flucloxacillin. Resistant *S. aureus* is more difficult and expensive to treat.

Box 21.5 Notifiable diseases in the UK

List of notifiable diseases to the CCDC under the Public Health (Infectious Diseases) Regulations 1988:

- Acute encephalitis
- Acute poliomyelitis
- Anthrax
- Cholera
- Diphtheria
- Dysentery
- Food poisoning
- Leptospirosis
- Malaria
- Measles
- Meningitis
- Meningococcal septicaemia (without meningitis)
- Mumps
- Ophthalmia neonatorum
- Plague
- Rabies
- Relapsing fever
- Rubella
- Scarlet fever
- Smallpox
- Tetanus
- Tuberculosis
- Typhoid fever
- Typhus fever
- Viral haemorrhagic fever
- Viral hepatitis
- Whooping cough
- Yellow fever
- Paratyphoid fever

Box 21.6 Infection risk labels

Label all specimens and request forms for patients from the following groups:

Hepatitis
Patients with possible viral hepatitis
Patients known to be hepatitis B or C positive
Jaundice in immunocompromised patients
Injecting drug users unless known to be blood borne virus negative

HIV Infection
All known HIV infected patients
All patients at high risk of HIV

Tuberculosis
Patients with known or suspected tuberculosis

'Exotic' infections
Patients with fever within 3 weeks of travel abroad
Patients known or suspected of having: typhoid, paratyphoid, brucellosis, malaria

> **Box 21.7** Control measures for MRSA
>
> • Ideally all patients should be isolated. When there are not enough isolation facilities, the ICT will advise if this is necessary
> • Special precautions are required (each hospital has guidance on the care of MRSA positive patients)
> • All healthcare staff, visitors and cleaners should be informed of the need for special precautions
> • A record should be made on the inside cover of the patient's notes: 'this patient has a history of colonisation/infection with MRSA'
> • Any receiving ward or department must be informed in advance of transfer
> • A history of MRSA infection or colonisation must be communicated in the TTO and discharge summary.

One-third of healthy people are colonised with *S. aureus* in their nose and skin (often the axillae and groins). Colonisation with MRSA in healthy people is not a problem, but in vulnerable patients it can progress to serious infection. Patients who are colonised with MRSA shed bacteria into the surrounding environment and pose a serious risk of cross infection. Healthcare staff may transfer MRSA between patients and become colonised themselves, especially if there is poor hand hygiene. Hand hygiene and a strict ward cleaning policy remain the most important measures to prevent the spread of infections including MRSA (Box 21.7).

Respiratory infections

Extra respiratory precautions are required for some alert conditions, for example multi-drug resistant pulmonary tuberculosis or pandemic influenza. A high-efficiency mask is used to protect against aerosol spread (these are close fitting with more dense material than normal theatre masks).

The Department of Health has published extensive guidelines on infection control and management of pandemic influenza [6]. Influenza is spread through droplets, direct and indirect contact. The following are measures which should be used in suspected cases of pandemic influenza:
• The patient should be isolated
• Staff should wear a gown or apron, gloves and high-efficiency mask
• Aerosol generating procedures such as tracheal intubation, bronchoscopy, chest physiotherapy require extra care (e.g. eye protection)
• This personal protective equipment must be changed immediately between patients
• The patient should wear a high-efficiency mask if travelling to other departments (e.g. radiology)
• Strict hand hygiene measures should be followed

- Respiratory secretions must be contained (e.g. if coughing or sneezing)
- The patient and visitors must be educated and follow these procedures.

Antibiotic prescribing

All doctors have a duty to prescribe antibiotics responsibly in order to curb the growth of antibiotic resistance. The following guidelines should be used:
- If the patient is well, locate the source of the infection before prescribing
- Use antibiotics only to treat bacterial infections
- Choose antibiotics which are active against the likely organism
- Send microbiological samples as a matter of routine before administering an antibiotic (e.g. urine, sputum, wound swabs, blood cultures)
- Follow local guidelines which incorporate data on local resistance patterns
- Change to more specific antibiotics when the results of microbiological tests are known
- Take alert infections into account, for example if a patient is colonised with MRSA and then develops sepsis, start an antibiotic that covers MRSA pending further results
- Do not hesitate to ask the ICT for advice.

Key points: Infection control

- HCAIs increase length of stay, morbidity and mortality and cost the NHS billions of pounds.
- 30% of HCAIs are preventable.
- Hand hygiene is the most important facet of infection control.
- Urinary catheters, peripheral cannulae and central lines should be removed as soon as they are no longer necessary.
- Alert organisms and alert conditions require special precautions.
- Antibiotics should be prescribed responsibly.

Exercises

Discuss the following:
- On the ward round, the consultant starts to enter the side room of a patient with *Clostridium difficile* without putting on gloves and an apron.
- After seeing the patient with *C. difficile*, the consultant uses only alcohol gel to clean his hands.
- Do you behave and dress in a way which facilitates infection control?
- Find out what your local pandemic influenza plans are, including the location of high-efficiency masks, and tell the rest of your department.
- A 68-year-old patient with diabetes and osteoarthritis is being admitted for a hip replacement. He was found to be MRSA colonised on routine swabs on his last admission 3 months ago. How will this affect his management?

References

1. National Institute of Clinical Excellence. *Infection Control, Prevention of Healthcare Associated Infection in Primary Care and Community Care*. National Institute of Clinical Excellence, London, 2003.
2. Emmerson AM, Enstone JE, Griffin M *et al.* The second national prevalence survey of infection in hospitals – overview of results. *Journal of Hospital Infection* 1996; **32**: 175–190.
3. Cooper NA, Forrest K and Cramp P. Practical procedures. In: *Essential Guide to Acute Care*, 2nd edn. Blackwells, Oxford, 2006.
4. Loh W, Ng V and Holton J. Bacterial flora on the white coats of medical students. *Journal of Hospital Infection* 2000; **45**: 65–68.
5. Department of Health. *Winning Ways: Working Together to Reduce Healthcare Associated Infection in England*. Department of Health, London, 2003. www.dh.gov.uk
6. British Thoracic Society, British Infection Society, Health Protection Agency. Clinical guidelines for patients with an influenza like illness during an influenza pandemic. www.dh.gov.uk pandemic flu pages.

CHAPTER 22

Use of evidence and guidelines

> **By the end of this chapter you will be able to:**
> - Understand the principles of evidence-based medicine
> - Understand absolute and relative risk
> - Know about different types of biomedical research papers
> - Know how to discuss evidence with patients
> - Understand how to use guidelines and protocols

Evidence-based medicine can be described as *one* part of a clinician's diagnostic and therapeutic tool bag, as illustrated in Fig. 22.1. Decisions about an individual patient's care do not rely on evidence alone, but on clinical expertise, the values and wishes of the patient and even whether a test or treatment is available. Doctors need both the best evidence and clinical expertise, as applying one without the other can be harmful.

Evidence-based medicine can be abused. 'Evidence' can be applied inappropriately or 'spun' on behalf of powerful interest groups such as drug companies. Therefore, it is important that all doctors understand the benefits and limitations of evidence-based medicine and how to interpret information from clinical trials for themselves.

Healthcare professionals require information all the time, but traditional sources of information are often out of date (e.g. textbooks) and doctors usually do not have the time it takes to keep up to date by reading journals. Only 2% of original articles in the biomedical journals are both valid and immediately clinically relevant. In the last 10 years access to information has improved with the development of systematic reviews, evidence-based journals which publish summaries of original articles, and information systems which allow us to find evidence at the touch of a button. Some well-known examples of these are:
- The Cochrane Library [1]
- Clinical Evidence [2]
- Drug and Therapeutics Bulletin [3]
- National Electronic Library for Health [4]

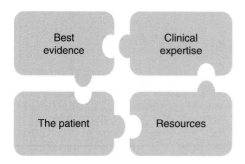

Figure 22.1 The role of evidence-based medicine.

- American College of Physicians (ACP) Journal Club [5]
- UpToDate [6].

Practising evidence-based medicine involves asking questions in your day-to-day clinical practice, taking time out to track down the evidence which answers those questions, critically appraising it, and putting the evidence in to practice.

Asking questions

Questions arise all the time in clinical practice, whether these are more general questions for novices or specific questions for experts. Questions can be related to history, examination, differential diagnosis, tests, treatments, prognosis or prevention. It is important to turn a clinical situation in to a clear, precise question so that this can be translated in to a search strategy and a useful answer.

Tracking down evidence

General questions for novices can easily be answered using textbooks or review articles. Review articles can be found using Medline or Google Scholar [7]. For more specific questions, the easiest way to track down evidence is to use a source such as one listed above which can be accessed on-line.

Part of your clinical training should include a training session in the medical library on how to perform a Medline search, since even the most experienced searchers miss many relevant articles. You can organise a session yourself with the librarian.

Critically appraising

Critical appraisal is the process by which a paper is studied and its main strengths and weaknesses are analysed. Many healthcare organisations hold journal clubs where critical appraisal is done during a team meeting. Most research papers are written in the 'IMRAD' format: introduction, methods, results and discussion. It is the methods section that is the most important in determining whether the results are valid.

When critically appraising a paper, ask yourself four broad questions:

1 What is the study about?
2 What type of study design has been used (e.g. randomised, blind, etc.)?
3 Are the methods used appropriate to the question?
4 What do the results really show?

> **Box 22.1** Making sense of numbers
>
> The effect of eating rhubarb on mortality:
>
> | Treatment | Total no | Dead | Alive |
> |---|---|---|---|
> | Eating rhubarb | 1000 | 200 | 800 |
> | Controls | 1000 | 400 | 600 |
>
> Rhubarb event rate (RER) = 200/1000 = 0.2
> Control event rate (CER) = 400/1000 = 0.4
>
> That is subjects who eat rhubarb have a 20% chance of dying and subjects who do not eat rhubarb have a 40% chance of dying.
>
> Absolute risk reduction = CER − RER or 0.4 − 0.2 = 0.2
>
> There is a 20% absolute risk reduction from eating rhubarb
>
> Relative risk reduction = (CER − RER)/CER or (0.4 − 0.2)/0.4 = 0.5
>
> There is a 50% relative risk reduction from eating rhubarb
> The numbers needed to treat with rhubarb to prevent one death is
> 1/ absolute risk reduction or 1/0.2 = 5.

Papers can be:
- Experiments (interventions in an artificial environment)
- Clinical trials (interventions in the context of clinical practice)
- Surveys
- Systematic reviews (summary of previous research using a predefined methodology)
- Meta-analyses (numerical data from more than one study is integrated).

Clinical trials involve a sample population, so the first question to ask is how was the sample chosen and how generalisable is this sample to my clinical practice? The research setting is also important. National studies with larger populations are more generalisable, compared with community-based studies which might be affected by local services or the environment. The sample size is also important as small numbers are unlikely to yield statistically significant results. Exclusion criteria gives useful information, as does the drop-out or refusal rate.

The sample population is compared to a control group. This can be a historical control or a contemporaneous one. However, the control group might introduce 'confounding variables' – a variable that itself affects the outcome. For example, if we wanted to compare the prevalence of menorrhagia in medical students compared to the general population and the control group included men that would be a confounding variable. To get around this, matched controls or random samples are chosen.

Results can be summarised in different ways. Raw numbers make more sense when expressed as proportions or probabilities (risk), as illustrated in Box 22.1 with pretend data.

Data can be presented in a way that makes an intervention sound much more clinically significant. For example, we know that the risk of deep vein thrombosis (DVT) is increased in women taking the combined oral contraceptive pill. Here is the same information presented in different ways:

- Risk of DVT five times higher in women taking the pill!
- Or you could say:
  - 5 in 100,000 women not taking the pill get a DVT each year
  - 25 in 100,000 women taking the pill get a DVT each year
  - This compares to 60 in 100,000 pregnant women who get a DVT each year.

Whilst the second explanation may be longer, it clearly conveys the low absolute risk of DVT in women taking the pill, even though the relative risk sounds high. Critically appraising is a practical exercise that is best learned through the exercises below, further reading and in the context of a journal club.

Different types of biomedical research papers

Different types of studies have different advantages and disadvantages. The main types of biomedical research papers are shown in Fig. 22.2.

Randomised controlled trials are thought to be the best way to do quantitative research, but like any other study design, they have advantages and disadvantages and may not be an appropriate way to answer certain questions.

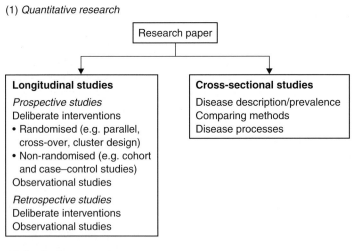

(1) *Quantitative research*

Research paper

Longitudinal studies

Prospective studies
Deliberate interventions
- Randomised (e.g. parallel, cross-over, cluster design)
- Non-randomised (e.g. cohort and case–control studies)
Observational studies

Retrospective studies
Deliberate interventions
Observational studies

Cross-sectional studies

Disease description/prevalence
Comparing methods
Disease processes

(2) *Qualitative research*

For example, naturalistic research, ethnographic studies

Using methods such as:
- Participant observation
- Interviews
- Study of documentary evidence

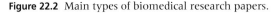

Figure 22.2 Main types of biomedical research papers.

In a randomised controlled trial the subjects are allocated randomly to different groups in parallel using a computer generated random number. The groups are followed for a certain time and analysed for specific outcomes (e.g. death, stroke). Randomisation ensures that the groups are similar, but even in these trials there can be hidden biases (e.g. exclusion criteria).

In a cross-over trial, less subjects are required because they receive both the intervention and the control, usually separated by a 'washout' period. In a cluster randomised trial, groups of subjects rather than individuals are randomised (e.g. general practices). A single blind trial means that the subjects did not know what intervention they received. A double blind trial means that the subjects and the investigators did not know what intervention each subject received.

Cohort studies are where groups are selected on the basis of differences in exposure to a certain intervention and then followed up to see what happens. The link between smoking and lung cancer was discovered this way. Case-control studies are when subjects are matched with a similar subject who does not have the characteristic in question.

Finally, well-designed qualitative research address questions (e.g. why?) that other research methods cannot, and is no less scientific.

Integrating evidence with clinical expertise

Use the exercise in Box 22.2 to practice a critical appraisal. The answers are at the end of this chapter.

Integrating evidence with clinical expertise involves taking what you know about the general treatment of a condition and putting it in the context of the patient in front of you. Having spent years at medical school learning the 'correct' treatment for various conditions, the reality is that patients often have contraindications, more than one problem that makes interventions more complicated, or beliefs and values that may have nothing to do with 'evidence'. Treatments have side effects which can sometimes be more important to patients than theoretical benefits. In addition, doctors are increasingly being asked to comment on 'evidence' from the Internet.

Box 22.2 An effective new treatment?

Effects of clopidogrel in addition to aspirin in patients with acute coronary syndromes without ST-segment elevation. *New England Journal of Medicine* 2001; **345(7)**: 494–502.

Imagine you are a geriatrician and you have been told about this effective new drug which you should be prescribing to all your patients with acute coronary syndromes. You decide to have a look at the original paper for yourself.

(*Continued p. 168*)

(*Continued.*)

The paper describes a randomised, double blind, placebo controlled trial. Patients with either electrocardiogram changes or a cardiac enzyme rise were allocated to receive aspirin plus clopidogrel or aspirin plus placebo within 24 hours of admission. Exclusion criteria included those on warfarin or contraindications to antiplatelet therapy. The outcomes of the study included death, myocardial infarction (MI) and bleeding complications. Over 12,000 patients were recruited.

The oldest patients in this study were 75 years old. The main results included:

- 582 out of 6259 patients in the intervention group died compared to 719 out of 6303 patients in the placebo group
- 324 out of 6259 patients in the intervention group went on to have a MI compared to 419 out of 6303 patients in the placebo group
- Major bleeding occurred in 231 out of 6259 patients in the intervention group compared to 169 out of 6303 patients in the placebo group.

Most major bleeds were gastrointestinal. Since only relative risk is quoted in the paper, work out the absolute risk reduction in death, MI and bleeding with and without clopidogrel and the numbers needed to treat for each outcome. Use Box 22.1 to help.

Having worked out these figures, decide for yourself whether there is evidence that this drug will benefit your patients. What are the issues raised by this paper? How is the data presented? Can you reduce the chances of harm from bleeding?

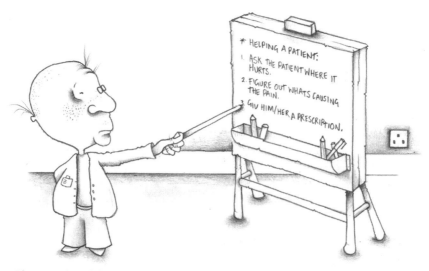

Evidence and guidelines.

Discussing evidence with patients

Discussing evidence with patients can be difficult. How can you translate the risks and benefits demonstrated in a population in a clinical trial to an individual? This is a particular problem when discussing prevention, for example the treatment of hypertension, when patients are being asked to take drugs to prevent a possible future event when they feel well.

Research shows that people find it hard to understand risk when presented in numerical terms [8]. Words such as 'common' or 'rare' mean different things to different people [9]. Risk can be described instead using visual scales or by comparing the chance of an event happening with things people more readily understand (e.g. winning the lottery). Individuals interpret risk in very different ways. An increased risk of a stroke might fill one person with dread but not necessarily another.

How you talk about risk also has an effect. Describing what people have to lose influences screening uptake more than describing what they have to gain. Emphasising the chance of survival rather than the chance of death makes people more likely to take treatment with risks. Information on relative rather than absolute risk is more persuasive (perhaps because people do not understand the difference) and patients become more wary the more information they are given [10].

Some patients prefer visual presentations of risk (bar charts, crowd figures) and an example is shown in Fig. 22.3. One way to discuss risk is to use a number of strategies over a period of time (booklets, videos, charts, question and answer sessions), particularly when discussing a risky intervention. However, people tend to perceive risk in a subconscious, subjective, personality dependent way rather than objectively basing their decisions on statistical data. You must be prepared for the question, 'What do *you* think doctor?'

Using guidelines and protocols

Common sources of guidelines are:
- National Institute for Clinical Excellence [12]
- Scottish Intercollegiate Guideline Network [13]
- National Service Frameworks [14]
- Royal Colleges
- Specialist societies
- Trust or departmental guidelines.

Guidelines and protocols can be useful tools for healthcare professionals, but they should not stop you from thinking (see Box 22.3).

Guidelines are systematically developed statements to assist healthcare professionals in their decision making. Guidelines do not take in to account specific clinical circumstances. The purpose of guidelines are to help [15]:
- Make evidence-based standards explicit
- Decision making in the clinic or at the bedside

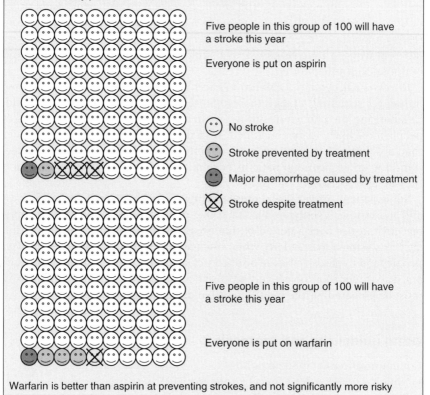

Primary prevention of stroke in non-valvular atrial fibrillation (AF) – aspirin or warfarin? [11]
- On no treatment, the risk of stroke is 5% per year in non-valvular AF
- The relative risk reduction with aspirin vs placebo is 24%
- The relative risk reduction with warfarin vs placebo is 62%
- The relative risk reduction with warfarin vs aspirin is 36%
- Warfarin is associated with risk of major haemorrhage per year in 0.9% people when compared with placebo
- When warfarin is compared with aspirin, the risk of major haemorrhage is similar

Note: Secondary prevention has different evidence

Five people in this group of 100 will have a stroke this year

Everyone is put on aspirin

No stroke

Stroke prevented by treatment

Major haemorrhage caused by treatment

Stroke despite treatment

Five people in this group of 100 will have a stroke this year

Everyone is put on warfarin

Warfarin is better than aspirin at preventing strokes, and not significantly more risky

Figure 22.3 Primary prevention of stroke in non-valvular AF.

- Provide a measure for assessing clinical performance
- Educate patients and professionals about best practice
- Improve cost effectiveness.

However, it is important to understand that guidelines do not replace clinical judgement about individual patients. Guidelines can be applied to the wrong clinical circumstances, can go out of date, or can be based on slim 'evidence' with which experts disagree. The inappropriate use of guidelines has been termed 'evidence-*biased* medicine' [16]. Guidelines are most effective when they have been developed locally, as part of an educational intervention, used in clinic or at the bedside [17]. It is good practice to document why guidelines

---

Box 22.3 Guideline warning!

A 30-year-old man was sent to hospital by his GP with a suspected pulmonary embolism. The patient had recently returned to the UK on a long-haul flight when he developed shortness of breath. He had a normal chest X-ray, electrocardiogram and blood tests. The pulmonary embolism protocol was followed, but because the protocol did not include long-haul flights as a risk factor for pulmonary embolism, the patient was categorised as low clinical probability for pulmonary embolism and discharged. His GP sent him back to hospital with a phone call and the patient was found to have a pulmonary embolism on computed tomography pulmonary angiography.

---

have not been followed in individual cases. This shows you have deliberately assessed the situation, rather than forgotten about it. As the saying goes, 'medicine begins where the protocol ends'.

Key points: Use of evidence and guidelines

- Evidence and clinical expertise are both required in the practice of medicine.
- Access to evidence has improved with the development of systematic reviews, evidence-based journals and information systems.
- 'Evidence' can be applied inappropriately or 'spun' on behalf of powerful interest groups such as drug companies.
- All doctors need to understand how to interpret information from clinical trials for themselves.
- Discussing evidence with patients can be difficult.
- Guidelines are to assist healthcare professionals in their decision making, not replace it.

Answers to the clopidogrel questions

Treatment	Total no	Dead	MI	Bleeding
Clopidogrel	6259	582	324	231
Placebo	6303	719	419	169

Death

Clopidogrel event rate (CER) = 582/6259 = 0.093
Placebo event rate (PER) = 719/6303 = 0.114
Absolute risk reduction = PER − CER = 0.021
Relative risk reduction = (PER − CER)/PER = 0.184
Numbers needed to treat to prevent one death is 1/absolute risk reduction = 48

Myocardial infarction

Clopidogrel event rate (CER) = 324/6259 = 0.052
Placebo event rate (PER) = 419/6303 = 0.067
Absolute risk reduction = PER − CER = 0.014
Relative risk reduction = (PER − CER)/PER = 0.212
Numbers needed to treat to prevent one death is 1/absolute risk reduction = 67

Bleeding

Clopidogrel event rate (CER) = 231/6259 = 0.037
Placebo event rate (PER) = 169/6303 = 0.027
Absolute risk reduction = PER − CER = −0.01
Relative risk reduction = (PER − CER)/PER = −0.37
Numbers needed to treat to cause one major bleed is 1/absolute risk = 100

Looking at the numbers needed to treat, for every 100 patients under the age of 75 years treated with clopidogrel, there are two less deaths, 1–2 less MIs and one major bleed.

Exercises

- Set up a journal club if you do not have one already. Use the four broad questions described above to critically appraise papers.
- Take one clinical decision that you or your team made this week. Find out on what evidence this decision was based.
- Think of a treatment or intervention about which you often advise patients. Is your explanation true to the evidence? What other ways of conveying risks vs benefits can you think of?
- Next time you attend a meeting sponsored by a drug company, make a note of how the results of a clinical trial are presented. If the trial was published in a peer reviewed journal, get a copy and examine it for yourself afterwards.

References

1. The Cochrane Library. www.thecochranelibrary.com
2. Clinical Evidence. www.clinicalevidence.com
3. Drug and Therapeutics Bulletin. www.dtb.org.uk/idtb
4. National Electronic Library for Health. www.nelh.nhs.uk
5. The American College of Physicians Journal Club. www.acpjc.org
6. UpToDate. www.uptodate.com
7. Google Scholar. http://scholar.google.com
8. Calman KC and Royston G. Personal paper: risk language and dialects. *British Medical Journal* 1997; **315**: 939–942.
9. Edwards A, Elwyn G and Mulley A. Explaining risks: turning numerical data into meaningful pictures. *British Medical Journal* 2002; **324**: 827–830.
10. Edwards AGK, Elwyn G, Matthews E and Pill R. Presenting risk information – a review of the effects of 'framing' and other manipulations on patient outcomes. *Journal of Health Communication* 2001; **6**: 61–82.

11. Review: anti-thrombotic agents prevent stroke in non-valvular atrial fibrillation. Evidence-based medicine 2000; **5**: 82. Patrick Pullicino (commentator).
12. National Institute for Clinical Excellence. www.nice.org.uk
13. Scottish Intercollegiate Guideline Network. www.sign.ac.uk
14. National Service Frameworks (Department of Health). www.dh.gov.uk/ PolicyAndGuidance/HealthAndSocialCareTopics/fs/en
15. Greenhalgh T. *How to Read a Paper. The Basics of Evidence Based Medicine*, 3rd edn. Blackwells, Oxford, 2006.
16. Edwards P, Jones S, Shale D *et al. Shared Care – A Model for Clinical Management.* Radcliffe Medical Press, Oxford, 1996.
17. Grimshaw JM and Russell IT. Effect of clinical guidelines on medical practice. A systematic review of rigorous evaluations. *Lancet* 1993; **342**: 1317–1322.

Further resources

- Bowers D, House A and Owens D. *Understanding Clinical Papers.* John Wiley & Sons, Chichester, 2001.
- Centre for evidence-based medicine. www.cebm.utoronto.ca
- Ismach RB. Teaching evidence-based medicine to medical students. *Academic Emergency Medicine* 2004; **11**: 1283. www.aemj.org
- Parker MJ. Managing an elderly patient with a fractured neck of femur. Evidence based case report. *British Medical Journal* 2000; **320**: 102–103.
- Sackett Dl, Strauss S, Richardson WS *et al. Evidence-Based Medicine. How to Practice and Teach EBM*, 2nd edn. Churchill-Livingstone, New York, 2000.

CHAPTER 23

Audit

By the end of this chapter you will be able to:

- Understand the context of audit in clinical governance
- Know the audit cycle
- Know the difference between audit and research
- Be able to perform an audit

Clinical audit is the process by which healthcare professionals regularly and systematically review their practice and, where necessary, change it. Clinical audit asks the question: 'Are we doing what we are meant to be doing?' Clinical audit can be large scale (e.g. a national audit on the management of myocardial infarction [1]) or small scale (e.g. how a department assesses older people with falls).

Participation in clinical audit is a requirement of all healthcare professionals. It is funded and supported by healthcare trusts and is an important part of clinical governance. Audit is a continual process, referred to as a cycle. Within the cycle are stages which establish what best practice is, measure delivery of care against explicit criteria, take action to improve care and monitor in order to sustain improvement. Clinical audit often involves multi-professional teams, including management.

The audit cycle

The audit cycle is represented diagrammatically in Fig. 23.1. For audit to be successful in promoting change, an organisation requires both a structure and a culture of audit. The different stages in audit are [2]:

- Choosing and preparing an audit
- Selecting audit standards
- Collecting data
- Making the case for improvements
- Sustaining improvements.

Choosing and preparing an audit

The focus of an audit project is those receiving care. The audit question should be simple. It is not appropriate to go and audit another department's practice without consent. Every doctor in training has to complete an audit project. It is worth making a note of things that interest or irritate you, as this can turn an

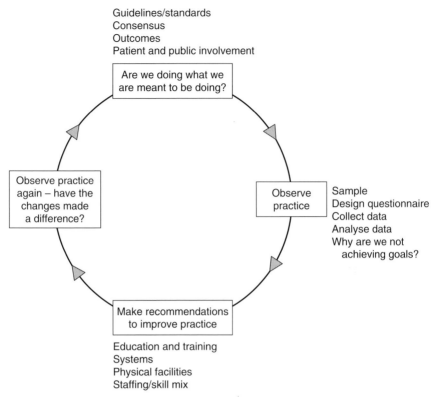

Guidelines/standards
Consensus
Outcomes
Patient and public involvement

Are we doing what we are meant to be doing?

Observe practice again – have the changes made a difference?

Observe practice

Sample
Design questionnaire
Collect data
Analyse data
Why are we not achieving goals?

Make recommendations to improve practice

Education and training
Systems
Physical facilities
Staffing/skill mix

Figure 23.1 The audit cycle.

audit into a tool for change rather than a dull compulsory project. The process of audit is also a way of learning skills such as project management, team work, questionnaire design, data collection, IT skills, presentational skills and change management. When you have a topic worth auditing, consider what is already known about the subject. What guidelines or consensus statements are there? What do patients think? You also need to choose an audit which you can complete in the time you have. Most hospitals have a clinical audit department. It is worth talking to the staff there to find out what support is available. Box 23.1 describes an example audit.

The standards selected for an audit project should be explicit and based on evidence. They should be clinically relevant and measurable. Standards can be related to the structure, process or outcome of care.

Collecting data
Data collection should be as simple as possible. Audit is concerned with clinical significance rather than statistical significance, so numbers and sampling are not as important as they are in research. Nevertheless, large (national) audit projects sometimes use some of the techniques used in research.

Box 23.1 An example audit

Two doctors had to complete an audit project. They discussed possible topics with senior colleagues and chose to audit how doctors assess older patients with recurrent falls. They chose the National Institute for Clinical Excellence (NICE) guidelines [3] as the standards and devised a simple checklist (yes or no) to ascertain whether the assessments were being done. Over 1 week, they had identified 30 patients admitted to hospital with recurrent falls and used the medical notes to assess whether the NICE guidelines were being followed.

They presented their findings to the departmental meeting. The audit found that the NICE guidelines were not being followed and some important aspects of the assessment were not being done at all. The presentation included an explanation of the guidelines and why they were important. Following this, the department devised a checklist which could be used on the admissions unit and incorporated guidelines into the new junior doctors' handbook. It was decided that the audit should be repeated in 6 months.

Assessment of older patients presenting with recurrent falls

Assessment	Performed?		
	Y	N	DK
Vision (acuity/cataracts)			
Lying + standing blood pressure			
Review of medication			
Get-up-and-go-test			
Neurological examination			
12-lead electrocardiogram			
Cardiovascular examination			
Referral to physiotherapy + occupational therapy			
Bone protection started			
Asked about incontinence			

Figure 23.2 Example audit data collection form.

Data for audit is most commonly gathered retrospectively from the Trust's records. The person collecting data for an audit should first design a data collection form. An example is shown in Fig. 23.2.

If more than one person is collecting data, they should all understand and agree on how to use the form, so that any confusing items are all recorded in the same way. It is often worth trying out the data collection form on a small number of cases first, to see if there are any obvious omissions that need to be addressed. A space for free text comments is often useful for obtaining valuable qualitative data. Patient confidentiality should be respected and all the audit data should be anonymised.

The information from the data collection form can be fed into a programme such as Microsoft Excel and presented in a simple fashion. Statistical analysis is not required for most audits.

Making the case for improvements

Feedback itself does not implement change. Educational materials, such as guidelines, also have little effect on their own. In order to successfully implement change based on audit, multifactorial interventions are more likely to be successful. Thinking in terms of the following categories can be useful:

• Barriers to change
• Education and training
• Systems
• Physical facilities
• Staffing/skill mix
• The involvement of the entire team, including management.

Making the case for change involves discussion and the communication and leadership skills described in Chapter 5. A well managed audit programme which addresses important questions, has sound leadership, an ethos of excellence with the patient at the centre and a supportive organisation, is far more likely to be successful in implementing sustained change.

Re-auditing

Re-auditing is a key component of the audit cycle to see whether the interventions which resulted from the initial audit have led to an improvement in standards. Very often, standards improve with each re-audit, but there is always room for improvement. An example of continuous improvement due to audit is the National Confidential Enquiry into Peri-operative Deaths (NCEPOD) (see Box 23.2).

The difference between audit and research

Audit and research are asking different questions, and the methodology used in audit is different to that of research. Audit is asking if we are doing what we are meant to be doing, whereas research asks the question, 'What *are* we meant to be doing?' The results of an audit are specific to a particular department or locality and not transferable to other healthcare settings in the way that research can be.

The differences between audit and research are illustrated in Box 23.3. It is important not to confuse the two when undertaking an audit project.

Box 23.2 National audit organisations

The Audit Commission is an independent public body which is responsible for ensuring that public money is spent efficiently and effectively in health and other public services. The Audit Commission promotes excellence as well as value for money. Two examples of Audit Commission reports are:

- Critical to success: the place of efficient and effective critical care services within the acute hospital. London 1999 (which led to the introduction of early warning scores and critical care outreach teams)
- United they stand: co-ordinating care for elderly patients with hip fracture. London 1995 (which promoted a co-ordinated orthogeriatric service).

The NCEPOD has now become part of the National Patient Safety Agency and has been renamed the National Confidential Enquiry into Patient Outcome and Death. It started life as a national audit of peri-operative deaths and its reports and recommendations have done much to improve patient safety. Examples of its recommendations include:

- That only life, limb or organ threatening surgery should take place after midnight
- That there should be dedicated acute theatres available 24 hours a day
- That all peri-operative patients should have thromboprophylaxis
- That all departments of surgery and anaesthesia should hold regular morbidity and mortality meetings.

Box 23.3 The difference between audit and research

Audit	Research
• Asks: Are we doing what we are meant to be doing?	• Asks: What are we meant to be doing?
• Aims to improve quality of care	• Aims to establish best practice
• Is specific to a particular setting	• Can be generalised to other settings
• Aims to improve services	• Aims to improve knowledge
• Is led by service providers	• Is led by researchers
• Is based on practice	• Is based on theory
• Never involves randomly allocating patients to different treatment groups	• May involve randomly allocating patients to different treatment groups
• Never involves a completely new treatment	• May involve a completely new treatment
• Deals with clinical significance	• Deals with statistical significance

Key points: Audit

- Clinical audit is how healthcare professionals regularly and systematically review their practice.
- Participation in audit is mandatory.
- Audit is a continual process with different stages, referred to as a cycle.
- Feedback alone does not implement change.
- Audit is not the same as research.

Exercises

- Discuss suitable topics for audit in your workplace.
- Perform an audit project using the process described above.
- Think back to an audit you have already performed. How could you make the case for change using multifactorial interventions. Think through the categories described.
- Have you seen examples where audit and research were confused?

References

1. Royal College of Physicians of London. *How Hospitals Manage Heart Attacks*. April 2002–March 2003. www.rcplondon.ac.uk/pubs/books/minap
2. National Institute for Clinical Excellence, Commission for Health Improvement, Royal College of Nursing, University of Leicester. *Principles for Best Practice in Clinical Audit*. Radcliffe Medical Press, Oxford, 2002.
3. National Institute of Clinical Excellence. *The Assessment and Prevention of Falls in Older People*. National Institute of Clinical Excellence guidance, London, 2003. www.nice.org.uk

PART IV
Teaching and Training

CHAPTER 24

Learning about learning

By the end of this chapter you will be able to:

- Know the qualities of a good teacher
- Understand the features of adult learning
- Know about some models of adult learning

All doctors are also teachers – of medical students, junior doctors, colleagues and other members of the healthcare team. The word 'doctor' comes from the Latin *docere* meaning 'to teach'. Teaching can be highly rewarding. Some people are naturally better teachers than others, but everyone can learn how to teach more effectively. It is a skill that can be developed and improved just like other skills.

Good teaching and learning

Recent changes in postgraduate medical education (Modernising Medical Careers and the introduction of the European Working Time Directive) mean that postgraduate training is becoming shorter and therefore more structured and focussed.

Good teaching requires time, some knowledge of adult learning and a varying degree of preparation. Teaching and learning are not the same thing. Many junior doctors when asked if they are taught reply, 'not much' but when asked if they *learn* reply, 'all the time!' Turn to the end of the chapter now, look at the exercises and think about teaching and learning you have experienced in the past.

From the exercises you will have developed some ideas of what you think makes a good teacher and a good learner. Good teachers tend to have the following four qualities: knowledge, interest, ability to communicate and respect for learners (see Box 24.1).

Learning is a two-way process and good learners require certain qualities as well. These include: engaging with the process, linking new information to prior knowledge and organising and accessing information. However, all of these attributes can be encouraged by a good teacher and a good learning environment.

Box 24.1 Qualities of a good teacher

- Knows the subject
- Can explain the subject
- Knows what resources are available
- Knows about the learners
- Can assess their own strengths and weaknesses
- Can respond to other people's comments
- Is enthusiastic about teaching and learning
- Has a good rapport with learners
- Can motivate the learners
- Can present information in different ways
- Can select appropriate materials
- Can provide variety in the lessons
- Wants to develop professionally.

Students do not want teachers who:

- Are always in a bad mood
- Are 'know-it-alls'
- Do not inspire respect
- Are always negative
- Are indifferent to teaching
- Show no passion for their subject
- Do not explain
- Make them feel anxious
- Are rude to them
- Are sarcastic.

Adult learners

It is generally considered that adults learn differently to children in many respects [1]. Adult learners:

- Have a motivation for learning
- Have the capacity to learn
- Are reflective – able to mull over ideas or facts
- Have clear goals and objectives (e.g. career progression).

Teachers need to bear in mind some of the features (or 'pillars') of adult learning when planning sessions:

- Adult learners are autonomous and self-directed. Teachers should actively involve them in the learning process, allow them to assume responsibility for presentations and group leadership, get their perspective on what topics to cover and act as a facilitator, guiding learners rather than supplying them with facts.

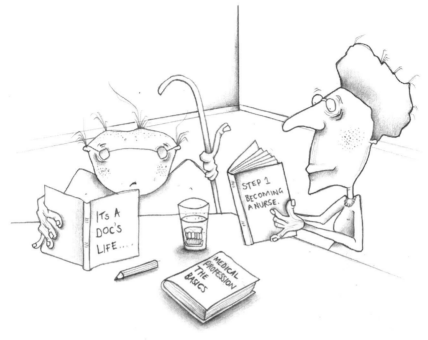

Adult learning.

- Adult learners have experience (e.g. work, family, previous education). They need to connect learning to their previous experience and knowledge. Teachers should draw out participants' experience and knowledge where relevant to the topic.
- Adult learners are goal orientated. Teachers should ensure that the programme is well organised, with clearly defined aims and objectives, and show how the teaching will help learners attain their goals.
- Adults are relevancy orientated. They need to see a reason for learning. It needs to be applicable to their work or other responsibilities to be of value. Teachers need to relate theories and concepts to familiar settings, and allow learners to choose projects that reflect their own interests.
- Adults are practical. They may not be interested in learning for its own sake. Teachers need to emphasise how learning can be put into practise.
- Adults learners want to be respected.

Models of adult learning

Various models of adult learning exist. All paint a different aspect of learning which can be helpful for teachers and learners alike.

Deep and superficial learning

You may have heard of the terms 'deep' and 'superficial' learning. Traditional teaching methods in schools encourage superficial learning. Superficial learners tend to want to get through a course and learn by reproducing. They study without reflection, memorise facts, treat each aspect of the course as unrelated chunks of knowledge and feel pressured by the amount of work involved.

Deep learners are interested in learning for its own sake and learn by relating ideas to previous knowledge. They look for patterns and underlying principles and adopt an evidence-based approach. However, deep learners may get side tracked at the expense of everything else they need to learn.

Deep learning is more likely to lead to long-term retention of knowledge and skills and the ability to apply learning to future problems. This is highly relevant to medicine. However, we all use different types of learning, sometimes at the same time, depending on the situation. For example, if you are on a ward round presenting a case you use the superficial approach to remember the patients name, age and presenting complaint. Deep learning occurs when you integrate the patient's diagnosis and treatment with previous knowledge and build up a database of knowledge about that complaint. As teachers, we can influence learning styles by encouraging deep learning. Questions asked of students can include more about concepts, ideas and decision making, rather than questions that emphasise rote learning such as, 'Tell me the seven causes of …'.

Domains of learning

The domains of learning were first described by Bloom [2] in the 1950s as the cognitive, psychomotor and affective domains. You may have heard these domains described in terms of knowledge, skills and attitudes. These are the broad divisions of any learning objective. For example, think about examining a patient. A student may have the knowledge to do it and have read about it in books – this is the cognitive domain. But examining a patient is also a practical skill – this is learning in the psychomotor domain. In addition, appropriate behaviour is required, for example not undressing the patient in public – this is the affective domain.

Traditionally, knowledge was the overriding domain that was taught at medical school. Practical skills were learned 'on the hoof' and new doctors had to look to their seniors for examples in the affective domain. Nowadays, these domains are emphasised and assessed as well. Box 24.2 illustrates more about each domain and how each has a hierarchy of learning objectives. The simplest behaviours are listed first, becoming more complex.

Knowing the different levels that learners need to move through in each domain can serve as a teaching aid and help to observe their progression. Miller's pyramid [3] is another way to look at the progression of learning within a specific objective. Miller's pyramid is more often used for the assessment process to examine which level a learner has reached (see Fig. 24.1).

Box 24.2 Domains of learning

Cognitive domain
- Knowledge: recognition and recall of information
- Comprehension: understanding information
- Application: uses information in context
- Analysis: separates into parts to reveal new relationships
- Synthesis: combines information to create a new situation
- Evaluation: reflects on judgement.

These six subdivisions can be reduced to recall of information, understanding and problem solving.

Psychomotor domain
- Imitation: observe skill and tries to reproduce it
- Manipulation: performs skill from instruction
- Precision: reproduces skill with accuracy and proportion
- Articulation: combines skills in sequence in harmony and consistently
- Naturalisation: completes skilful tasks competently and automatically.

Remember learning to drive? Teaching a skill is discussed further in Chapter 28.

Affective domain
- Receiving: listening
- Responding: response to a stimuli when expected
- Valuing: displays behaviour consistent with a single belief without coercion
- Organising: shows commitment to a set of values by behaviour
- Characterising: behaviour consistent with a value system.

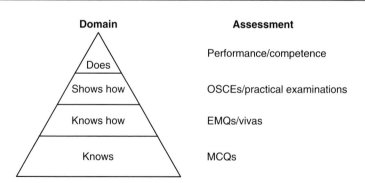

Miller's pyramid describes levels of learning and implies that a learner should have a 'knowledge base' in order to be able to perform a task competently.

OSCE: objective structured clinical examination
EMQs: extended matching questions
MCQs: multiple choice questions

Figure 24.1 Miller's pyramid.

Learning styles

In the 1980s, Kolb developed a four-stage cycle model to explain how adults learn a skill [4]. In effect, Kolb's learning cycle says that effective learning occurs when we get involved in a learning experience (concrete experience), have to think about the experience (reflective observation), theorise and assimilate this with what we already know (abstract conceptualisation) and practice or experiment with this new knowledge (active experimentation). His idea was that learning is a process and that effective learning occurs when people spend time in each part of the cycle. Applying this to medicine, 'see one, do one' becomes 'see one, think about one, do one, reflect on one and try again'.

The observation that people tend to spend more time in some steps of this cycle rather than others led to the concept of learning styles, expanded by Honey and Mumford [5]. Fig. 24.2 illustrates these two models.

In Kolb's model, the vertical axis represents how people think about things, and the horizontal axis represents how people like to do things. Four main learning styles are apparent:

1 People that like to feel and watch
2 People that like to think and watch
3 People that like to think and do
4 People that like to feel and do.

Fig. 24.3 summarises the characteristics of the different learning styles and activities that support each learning style.

Everyone can adopt any teaching or learning style. What this model does is help teachers to be aware that differences exist. Being able to change teaching styles has the advantage of engaging more learners and can also be used to change the tempo of a session and increase attention. Even though we tend to teach in our preferred learning style, it is better to teach enthusiastically in your own style rather than adopt another one awkwardly.

How professionals learn

Einstein said 'knowledge is experience – everything else is just information.' Medical education is a complex process and it takes time to build new knowledge onto existing knowledge before it finally makes sense. Learning occurs through repetition and mistakes. As teachers, we should not expect every learner to 'get it' first time around, but instead encourage repetition and different aspects of the learning cycle.

Learning is best conceived as a process rather than an outcome. A knowledge base is required in medicine which sets the 'stage' for problem solving, but time and experience along with feedback is extremely important when it comes to developing expert professional practice [6], which is something more than simply outcome-based learning.

Student-centred learning

Previously, teachers would impart knowledge to adult learners who were considered empty vessels waiting to be filled. Many institutions existed on this

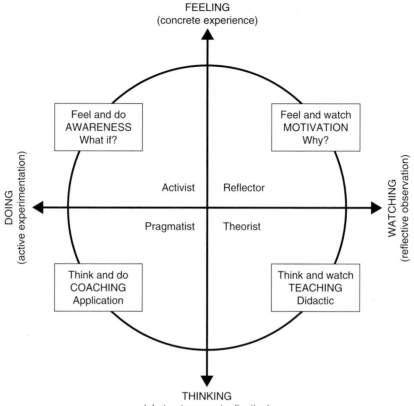

In this diagram, the cycle represents the process of learning. For example, imagine you are given the task of teaching a small group of doctors how to perform a lumbar puncture. The cycle helps to explain the process that learners need to go through in order to learn successfully. This process need not start at any point, but includes theory, coaching (which could include simulation), 'real life' activity and reflection.

At every stage, there will be people who prefer to learn in a certain way. Some will prefer theory whereas others will prefer practice. The reality is they need all stages to learn effectively. This model can be applied to almost any subject, not just practical procedures.

Figure 24.2 The learning cycle and learning styles.

concept and the learner was no more than a passive observer. If learning did not take place, it was the fault of the learner. With increased knowledge about adult learning, and medical education in particular, a more student-centred approach to teaching and learning is developing. This approach requires that teachers as well as learners have certain attributes.

Teachers should:

- Ensure integration across the curriculum
- Use the enquiry process

Learning style	Characteristic strengths of each learning style	Activities that support that learning style	Activities as a teacher with that learning style
People who like to feel and watch (reflectors)	Imaginative ability and generation of ideas	Investigations and puzzles Reading and essay writing Use of the library, factual research Lectures Tests	Acts as a transmitter to further students within the discipline
People who like to think and watch (theorists)	Creating theoretical models and making sense of disparate observations	Problem solving Role-playing Making and constructing Writing for an audience Wide variety of media (e.g. video, internet, music)	Acts as a manager to prepare students to perform the skills in the real world
People who like to think and do (pragmatists)	Practical application of ideas	Group work Broad brief with choices Presentations Opportunity to make mistakes	Acts as a colleague to enhance the students vision of what could be achievable
People who like to feel and do (activists)	Carrying out plans and tasks that involve them in new experiences	Debate Conversations Structured group work Peer teaching and learning Opportunities to hypothesise, ask questions and use imagination	Acts as facilitator to further student growth and development

Figure 24.3 How different learning styles like to learn and teach.

- Be a mentor and a guide
- Be flexible
- Be enthusiastic.
  Students should:
- Take responsibility and an active role
- Make their own choices about when and how to learn
- Be interested and curious.

Making learning happen

Learning is not necessarily a process that occurs in discrete domains and stages. Different models can be used at different times, depending on the situation and

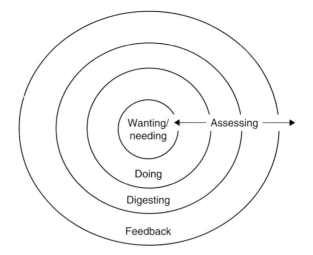

The five factors underpinning successful learning all affect each other and occur simultaneously, rather like ripples on a pond, bouncing backwards and forwards, and interacting with each other. Assessment can be applied to all these factors.

Reproduced with permission by Phil Race. Five factors underpinning successful learning. In: *Making Learning Happen*. SAGE Publications, London, 2005.

Figure 24.4 Ripples on a pond.

the learner. In a simple model, Race describes five factors which are essential for successful adult learning [7]. These are:

1 Wanting to learn (intrinsic motivation)
2 Needing to learn (extrinsic motivation)
3 Learning by doing (practice, repetition, experience)
4 Making sense of things, or digesting (rather than just storing information)
5 Learning through feedback.

All of these factors occur simultaneously and affect each other, like ripples on the surface of a pond (see Fig. 24.4). As teachers we can address these factors simultaneously as well.

'Assessment drives learning' is an accepted fact in educational circles. So if you want learners to know something, assess it. Think of your own experience. You have probably worked hard at learning something because it was going to be tested in some way. Assessment has the advantage of encouraging learning, but sometimes the disadvantage of encouraging strategic learning at the expense of deep, or more relevant learning. Strategic learning at times is not necessarily a bad thing. Teachers should also strategically teach (e.g. when asked to teach for a postgraduate examination, using examination questions rather than giving a lecture).

Finally, both teachers and learners need aims and objectives. This helps learners to have a mental framework in which to store knowledge. It also focuses the mind of the teacher – at the end of this programme, what should these learners be able to know and do?

Key points: Learning about learning

- All doctors are teachers.
- Good teaching requires time, knowledge of adult learning and preparation.
- Adults learners have certain characteristics.
- Questions about concepts, ideas and decision making encourage deep learning.
- Learning occurs in different domains.
- Understanding different models of learning helps the process of teaching.
- Expert professional practice develops with time, experience and feedback.
- Assessment drives learning.

Exercises

- We can all remember teachers who inspired us. What were the qualities of teachers that inspired you?
- Think of a teacher in your medical training that you disliked. What was it about that teacher that you disliked?
- Think of a colleague or colleagues that you like teaching. Why do you enjoy the experience?
- Think of a trainee that you have problems teaching. What is it about the individual that you think causes the problem?

References

1. Knowles M. *Self-directed Learning*. Follet, Englewood Cliffs, New Jersey, 1975.
2. Bloom BS. *Taxonomy of Educational Objectives*. Allyn and Bacon, Boston, MA, 1984.
3. Miller GE. The assessment of clinical skills/competence/performance. *Academic Medicine* 1990; **65**: S63–S67.
4. Kolb DA. *Experiential Learning – Experience as the Source of Learning and Development*. Prentice-Hall, Englewood Cliffs, New Jersey, 1984.
5. Honey P and Mumford A. *The Manual of Learning Styles*. Peter Honey, Maidenhead, 1982.
6. Talbot M. Good wine may need to mature: a critique of accelerated higher specialist training. Evidence from cognitive neuroscience. *Medical Education* 2004; **38**: 399–408.
7. Race P. *Making Learning Happen: A Guide for Post-compulsory Education*. Sage, London, 2005.

CHAPTER 25

Teaching large groups

By the end of this chapter you will be able to:

- Plan and deliver a lecture
- Devise a lesson plan for teaching a large group
- Know how to introduce interactivity into lectures

Lectures fell out of favour in the 1990s as a teaching method in undergraduate medicine when it was realised that they are an inadequate way to teach skills, attitudes and higher-order thinking. However, lectures are still effective in [1]:

- Teaching large groups
- Providing core knowledge
- Demonstrating enthusiasm of teachers for their subject
- Directing learning.

A traditional lecture encourages passivity, as this definition captures – 'lecture: the process by which the notes of the professor become the notes of the student without ever passing through the mind of either'. Research on lectures as an educational tool shows that the attention of students is highest for the first 10 minutes, then quickly falls before rising slightly before the end [1]. If a change in delivery or interactivity is introduced, attention rises again but never quite reaches the initial peak. Fig. 25.1 illustrates this.

You have been asked to deliver a lecture to medical students – what should you do? Before any teaching episode you must ask three questions of the person requesting your help:

- Who am I teaching? (e.g. medical students, nursing staff or senior house officers)
- What do they already know? (e.g. is this teaching part of a course)
- What do you want me to teach? (e.g. what are the aims and objectives of this session)

Similarly, if you are planning an educational programme, this is important information to impart to individual teachers.

Even before you start to plan the educational content of a lecture, there are important logistics to consider: the venue, how many students will be there and what audio-visual equipment is provided. If you can, try and visit the lecture theatre beforehand to familiarise yourself with the equipment so you and the students can concentrate on the educational content. Sometimes, even

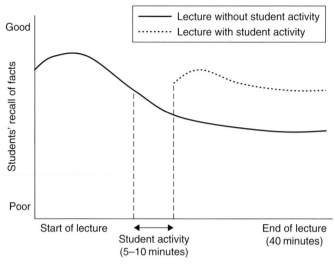

Figure 25.1 Attention in lectures.

Box 25.1 Lack of preparation?

One of the authors was asked to lecture 80 medical students. She was told the venue and had never been there before, so she went the day before to check the facilities, load her presentation and prepare handouts. The next day she arrived at the lecture theatre in good time but knew something was wrong as the lecture theatre was empty. She had been told the wrong venue, which was in the building next door. She made it in time and had a back up of her talk to reload on to the computer. On entering the lecture theatre she got another shock as there were 240 medical students, not 80 as she had been told. Handouts had to be shared!

---

with the best preparation, things can still go wrong (see Box 25.1) so always have a back-up plan.

Planning a lecture

When planning any teaching episode you must consider [2]:
- The environment (lighting, temperature, acoustics and seating)
- The set (establishing the mood, aims and objectives)
- The dialogue (the main body of teaching)
- Closure (summary and questions).

It may sound obvious, but as a teacher you are responsible for ensuring that the lighting, temperature, acoustics and seating are all conducive to learning.

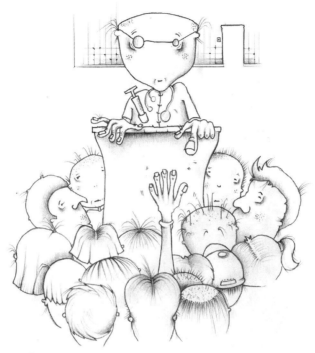

Large group teaching.

All teaching episodes should start with an outline or list of objectives. If you do not tell the learner the aims and objectives of the session they will find it hard to follow the whole process. For the learner, this is like solving a jigsaw puzzle without seeing the picture. The next step is to deliver information. There are many different ways of doing this. One can look at things systematically, tell a story or state a problem and provide an answer. At the end you should provide a summary of what you have said.

In other words, tell your audience what you are going to tell them, tell them, and then tell them what you just told them. Presentation issues such as the use of PowerPoint are discussed in Chapter 27.

During a lecture *you must speak slowly and clearly and face the audience.* Wear comfortable clothes. Only very experienced lecturers can operate without a script. Most people need to have their talk written out in front of them which they can refer to as they go along. Rehearsal is important. Ask a colleague if they will listen to you practice.

A useful exercise for any educational episode is to plan it on paper as a lesson plan. Your lesson plan should include the aims and objectives, timings for each section of the lecture and which equipment you will be using for that section. Figs 25.2 and 25.3 show example lesson plans.

Lecture: physiology and pharmacology of pain
Aims: understanding the physiology and pharmacological treatment of pain

Timing (min)	Teacher activity	Student activity	Resources
5	Introduction Definition Assessment	Listening	PowerPoint
10	Introduce the stickman and ask the students in buzz groups to draw the pain pathways on it	Buzz groups	Paper stick man
5	Get back answers from the groups	One student at the front filling in flip chart, the others providing the answers	Flip chart
15	The introduction of analgesic drugs	Listening	PowerPoint
10	On the paper stickman draw were the analgesic drugs work	Buzz groups	Paper stickman
5	Get back answers from the groups	One student at the front filling in flip chart, the others providing the answers	Flip chart
5	Summary Questions	Questions	Handout Filled in stickman Analgesic ladder

Figure 25.2 Example lesson plan A.

Handouts are good for summaries, homework and further reading. Although many lecturers do not like giving out handouts at the start of a lecture, students prefer this. They still listen to what you are saying. The handout provides a structure and room for notes.

How to introduce interactivity into a lecture

There are many ways to introduce interactivity to a lecture:
• Divide students into 'buzz groups', for example two students turn around to speak with the two students behind them. Ask the groups to address a question or problem on the screen. If the groups feed back, there is 'safety in numbers' so no one feels intimidated.
• Put up a question in the middle of the presentation that needs working out. For example, in a lecture on local anaesthesia ask students to work out doses for theoretical patients.

Workshop: opportunistic clinical teaching
Aims: to improve understanding of what makes good opportunistic clinical teaching

Timing (min)	Teacher activity	Student activity	Resources
5	Introduction	Listening	
10	What you are hoping to get from the workshop?	Participating	
15	Background to clinical teaching	Listening	PowerPoint
15	What challenges/ problems have you faced concerning clinical teaching?	Buzz groups	
15	Feed back to large group	Participating	Flip charts
10	What the literature says	Listening	PowerPoint
10	Break	Break	
15	What have you seen that addresses these challenges/problems?	Buzz groups	
15	Feed back to large group	Participating	Flip charts
10	What the literature says	Listening	PowerPoint
5	Summary/close	Take away literature pack Evaluation forms	

Figure 25.3 Example lesson plan B.

- Ask for answers to multiple choice questions (MCQs) on the screen by a show of hands or electronic voting consoles. This is a good way of establishing whether students have understood the teaching so far.
- Change the media you are using. Move from PowerPoint to a flip chart or video.
- Build exercises into your handout.

Sometimes large groups are not the best forum for questions as students may feel intimidated to speak up. One way around this is to announce that you will stay behind at the end to take questions. Another is to ask for written questions to be forwarded during a break – that way you can select particular questions to address.

Research about what students liked in lectures shows that they appreciated [3]:

- Material pitched at the right level
- Clear structure
- Appropriate pace
- Enthusiasm

- Ability to provide good explanations
- Variety and interactivity.

Giving good lectures is not easy but does get better with practice. For experienced lecturers interactivity can feel less controlled than the traditional way of reading out slides to a passive group. However, we have to remember that the point of a lecture is so that people can learn.

Key points: Teaching large groups

- Lectures are good for providing core knowledge and directing learning.
- Before giving a lecture there are important practical facts you need to know.
- A lecture consists of environment, set, dialogue and closure.
- Lecturers must speak slowly and clearly, and face the audience.
- Interactivity during lectures increases attention.

Exercises

- In the next lecture you attend, make a note of whether the lecturer has used the structure of set (aims and objectives), dialogue and closure (summary and questions).
- Did the lecturer speak slowly and clearly?
- Think about how you can introduce some interactivity into a lecture you might give.

References

1. Bligh D. *What's the Use of Lectures?* Intellect Books, Exeter 2002.
2. Mackway-Jones K and Walker M (eds). *Pocket Guide to Teaching for Medical Instructors.* BMJ Books, London, 1999.
3. Ramsden P. *Learning to Teach in Higher Education*. Routledge, London, 1992.

Further resources

- Brown S and Race P. *Lecturing: A Practical Guide*. Kogan Page, London, 2002.
- Race P (ed.). *2000 Tips for Lecturers*. Kogan Page, London, 1999.

CHAPTER 26

Teaching small groups

By the end of this chapter you will be able to:

- Understand the educational principles in teaching small groups
- Know when to use small group teaching
- Understand what makes a good facilitator

Running small groups looks easy. Junior doctors are much more likely to have been a member of a small group rather than a facilitator. However, have you been invited or instructed to run a tutorial for a small group at short notice? Would you have given a lecture to 200 people with the same notice on the same topic?

Small group teaching should come with a hazard warning. On the one hand, the group facilitator may find it difficult to predict how a group of individuals will interact or react. The facilitator is leaping into the unknown each time he starts with a new group. On the other hand, learners might feel uncomfortable or threatened because in a small group there is nowhere to hide or sleep. However, they might even learn or have fun.

It is tempting to compare and contrast small group teaching to lectures. An equivalent starting point is the characteristics of ideal adult learners as described in Chapter 24. The key points to remember are that adult learners:

- Learn effectively when an episode is meaningful and active
- Need to become autonomous
- Need constructive feedback
- Learn best when learning is experience centred
- Require time for reflection
- Need clear goals and objectives.

We could then proceed to make a list of how different types of teaching methods match the characteristics of an adult learner. While neither lecturing nor teaching small groups meets every characteristic, the key to planning teaching is to fit the educational method to the needs of the learner, not to fit the learner in to the educational method chosen by the teacher.

What makes small group teaching different to lectures? One of the obvious differences is the size of the group. However, you do find teachers giving lectures to small numbers of people and some lectures are very interactive. The main difference is that small group teaching requires active participation

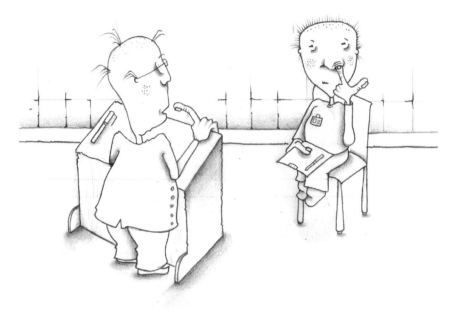

Small group teaching.

and collaboration by all present and often the production or completion of a task.

What is a small group?

We work in clinical small groups in theatre, on the ward, in outpatients and in general practice. Generally, the acceptable size of a small group for teaching purposes is somewhere between 5 and 12 people. With fewer or more people than this, the ways in which the members of the group interact makes the small group function differently. Therefore, for the rest of this chapter, these numbers will form the working definition of a small group.

Small groups sessions have a variety of titles: seminars, tutorials, closed discussions, open discussions and workshops. Have you been to one of these small group teaching sessions only to experience a lecture? In a small group the teacher's role is to facilitate learning through discussion. The role is not just to convey information but also to help the understanding of it.

Small group teaching is a way of 'teaching' that requires the collaboration of all those taking part, leading to a broader and hopefully deeper learning episode. Small group teaching works well for parts of the curriculum that require synthesis and evaluation of knowledge and where students can discuss in a group their understanding of concepts. However, small group teaching also helps to foster other generic skills that are very relevant to medicine: communication,

> **Box 26.1** Advantages to learners in small group teaching
>
> - Active participation
> - Development of independence and maturity
> - Facilitators can check students' understanding of subjects
> - Learners can think critically and systematically
> - Easier to deal with difficult subject matter
> - Fostering the ability to work in teams
> - Instant feedback
> - Students can ask questions that they feel unable to ask in lectures
> - Students can learn from each other
> - It is student-centred learning
> - It is a good place for tutors to role model attitudes.

leadership and co-operation. Another benefit of small group teaching is socialisation. Some students like to know how they are doing compared with others. There is nothing as good as finding out that you are not stupid and the rest of the class has been struggling to understand a concept as well. Box 26.1 lists the advantages to the learner of small group teaching.

The two main types of small group are known as closed (convergent) or open (divergent). These will be discussed in more detail below. It is important to understand the principle differences between these because they function very differently and inappropriate selection can lead to serious difficulties.

Closed discussions

In closed discussions, the facilitator maintains control throughout the session. All interactions take place through the facilitator. It can be compared to a well-run committee meeting where all discussion passes through the chairperson. This is achieved by careful attention to the layout of the room, classically in a horseshoe with each of the learners equally spaced. The facilitator sits or stands in the middle so that he can see and interact with all the learners. This arrangement makes it quite difficult for conversations to spring up between the participants, and deliberately so. Closed questions by the facilitator, that is those with a right or wrong answer, help retain control.

The closed discussion is effective when the planned intention of the teaching session is:
- To impart new knowledge
- To revise what should already be known
- A definitive answer to posed questions
- A need to control time.

Examples of topics that might be included in a closed discussion are:
- How to manage a 'blue' patient
- The role of pulse oximetry

- The theoretical management of cardiac arrest
- The options available for post-operative pain relief.

Open discussions

Open discussions are altogether different, although they appear similar to a closed discussion. When conducted by an expert, an open discussion can look much easier than a closed discussion. But beware!

The intention of an open discussion is that while the discussion may focus towards a specific question, the direction that the discussion will follow is unknown. Open discussions are dangerous because the technique encourages and even requires the participants to share their own opinions. There is no longer the safety net of having right or wrong answers. An example of this might be an open discussion about whether those over 80 years old should have cardiopulmonary resuscitation. This discussion could get out of control. A group member might have an elderly relative who was successfully resuscitated yesterday, whereas others may have strong opposing views.

However, despite these potential difficulties open discussions are a powerful way of helping learners to work with a group, to put together coherent arguments and to learn to listen to others' points of view. It can be used as a way of demonstrating how others think and what acceptable behaviour is.

In order to facilitate this level of discussion the format of the group is different. While there is a leader to focus and guide the discussion, all members of the group need to have the opportunity to participate equally. They need to be at the same height, equally spaced in a circle. This allows everyone to see and speak to everyone else in the group. The facilitator forms part of the circle. Managing this sort of discussion is much more difficult than in a closed group and time keeping can be a problem, especially with the use of open questions, which have no 'right' answer.

The open discussion works effectively when the planned intention of the teaching session is to help learners learn:
- To discuss a topic constructively
- To listen to others
- To function within a group
- From each other.

The sort of topics that might be included in an open discussion are:
- What constitutes informed consent?
- How cost influences treatment
- The value of 4-month rotations in Foundation training
- Ethical issues.

Other ways of running small groups include buzz groups, brain-storming, 'fish bowling' (where one group discusses in a circle and the other group observes) and 'snowballing' (where small groups feedback to larger and larger groups). These are all methods to increase group interaction. See Fig. 26.1 for the different seating arrangements for closed and open discussion groups.

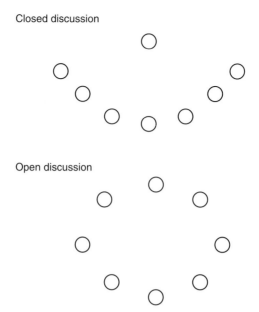

Figure 26.1 Seating arrangements for types of small group discussions.

Facilitation

Closed and open discussions require a facilitator. Good facilitators make it look easy. The facilitator may or may not be a content expert. Many medical schools run groups with two facilitators whose knowledge compliments each other's, for example a clinician and a scientist. It still requires as much preparation to facilitate a small group as giving a lecture – for the first time, plan roughly 4 hours preparation for every 1 hour tutorial. The amount of work and skill required is often underestimated. Preparations include the environment, set, dialogue and closure (as discussed in Chapter 25), course reading material and prop preparation.

The facilitator sets the agenda and focuses the group on the issues. A good facilitator has the following qualities so the small group session runs smoothly:
- Competence and commitment
- Relaxed, interested and organised
- Maintains contact with learners – expert use of body language
- An active and expert listener
- A motivator
- Creates equal opportunities for all
- Pays attention to the self-esteem of all
- Has the ability to summarise what people say, rephrasing 'incorrect' and emphasising 'correct'
- Is non-judgemental.

> **Box 26.2** Problems with small group teaching
>
> - Weak students may become discouraged
> - Bright students may become bored
> - Some discussions may be irrelevant
> - Different opinions may lead to arguments
> - Talkers can monopolise time and attention
> - The tutor gives a lecture rather than facilitates
> - The tutor takes over and leads the discussion
> - Lack of interaction from some students
> - Lack of preparation by students
> - Logistics – it requires more tutor time, more rooms and resources.

- Uses questions carefully
- Can give positive feedback.

There are different ways in which facilitators can function:

- Chairperson – task centred (closed discussion)
- Facilitator – process centred (open discussion)
- Instructor – skill station
- Participant – no leader
- Devil's advocate – counter arguments
- Agitator – dislikes comfortable discussion.

While the first three functions work well it is best to avoid the last two functions. It is not unusual to face these spontaneously from group members. Box 26.2 illustrates some of the problems that can be encountered when facilitating small groups.

Opportunistic clinical teaching

Opportunistic clinical teaching is a type of small group teaching in which students experience real life clinical situations and integrate all domains of learning: knowledge, skills and attitudes. Opportunistic clinical teaching occurs during ward rounds, in outpatient clinics, in general practice and in operating theatres (see Box 26.3). Teachers often find this kind of teaching difficult, as the competing demands of patients and trainees sometimes conflict. However, 'opportunistic' does not mean that planning cannot be done. With planning this form of teaching can be very beneficial.

Always have an aim in mind when beginning a teaching session – many teachers waffle about a pet topic that is not relevant to the student. Use questions to check understanding. End the session by asking the student to do homework about the subject you have taught and to present this next time you meet.

As with any form of teaching it is the teacher's knowledge, skills and enthusiasm that matter most.

Box 26.3 Opportunistic teaching

A stressed physician wondered how he could do the post-take ward round and teach a medical student, house officer and two senior house officers (SHOs) at the same time. Rather than feeling under pressure to talk about every case, he decided to focus on one medical topic for the morning. The team agreed on the topic of electrocardiogram (ECG) interpretation. At the end of the ward round, the physician gave feedback and directed the trainees towards further resources for learning.

Key points: Teaching small groups

- Small group sessions have a variety of titles: seminars, tutorials, discussions and workshops.
- Small group teaching requires active participation, collaboration and often the production or completion of a task.
- The two main types of small group teaching are known as closed (convergent) or open (divergent).
- Small group teaching requires the teacher to be a facilitator.
- Opportunistic clinical teaching can be planned in advance.

Exercises

- Think about your current experience of small group teaching. Is there active participation, collaboration or a task involved?
- Think about the Foundation Programme teaching sessions you have experienced. Is the teaching interactive? Does it correlate with what you know about adult learning?
- Look at Box 26.1 (advantages to learners in small group teaching) and Box 26.2 (problems with small group teaching). Have you experienced any of these? How do you think a facilitator could deal with some of the problems listed?

Further reading

- Harris D, Peyton R and Walker M. *Training the Trainers: Learning and Teaching*. Royal College of Surgeons, London, 1996.
- Jaques D. *Learning in Groups: A Handbook for Improving Group Work*. Kogan Page, London, 2000.
- Jaques D. Teaching in small groups. *British Medical Journal* 2000; **326**: 492–494.

- Mackway-Jones K and Walker M. Pocket Guide to Teaching for Medical Instructors. BMJ Books, London, 1999.
- McGill I and Beaty L. *Action Learning: A Guide for Professional, Management and Educational Development*. Kogan Page, London, 1995.
- Peyton R. *Teaching and Learning in Medical Practice*. Manticore, Guildford, 1998.
- Walton H. Small group methods in medical teaching. *Medical Education Book 1*, ASME, Dundee, 1973.
- Weinstein K. *Action Learning: A Practical Guide*, 2nd edn. Gower, Aldershot, 1999.

CHAPTER 27

Presentations

By the end of this chapter you will be able to:

- Give effective presentations
- Plan a workshop
- Plan and present a poster

Presentations are different from lectures. Presentations take place at lunchtime meetings, journal clubs, conferences and interviews. A chairperson is usually present to keep time. The audience can be very mixed, including senior colleagues who are more experienced than you, peers and people from other disciplines who may not know some of the basics – and you want to impress them all.

During a presentation, the audience is not necessarily present in order to be 'taught'. Rather, they wish to be informed of your thoughts, research and conclusions. Challenging questions can be asked of you. Nevertheless, there are lots of similarities between lectures and presentations including planning, the use of technology and controlling your nerves.

Usually, a presentation is on something you have spent a lot of time researching and you may have a lot to say. Part of the art of presentations is in deciding what information should and should not be presented. What is your main message? Can you point interested people towards further resources? The answer is *not* to speak faster in order to cram every piece of information in, or use tiny font on the overhead projector.

Features of effective presentations include the following.

Delivery
- Keeping to time
- Speaking slowly, clearly and audibly
- Facing the audience rather than the screen
- Making sure the slide or overheads are legible
- Not just reading out your slides
- Using laser pointers sparingly
- Making sure you know your equipment.

Content
- Being clear and concise
- Structuring your presentation with an obvious beginning, middle and end.

It can be helpful to get a friend to watch you run through your presentation, using these points as a guide. It is amazing how many of us give presentations whilst turned away from the audience, or using font that is difficult to read, or merely reading out what is on the slides. The point of audio–visual aids such as PowerPoint or transparencies is to supplement the presentation, not *be* the presentation.

How we put our message across is as important as what we have to say. There are three elements to face to face communication, known as the '7%-38%-55% rule' [1]:

- Words 7%
- Tone of voice 38%
- Body language 55%.

These figures were derived from experiments dealing with communication of feelings and attitudes and convey the importance of non-verbal communication.

Practice looking confident and smiling at the audience. Someone will always smile back even if the audience are complete strangers (try this, it really does work) and this will help you relax and look more confident. Memorise the first 30 seconds of your presentation so as not to look down at your prompts too early. Speak so slowly that it feels strange to you. We all speak faster than we should, partly because of nerves, and sometimes due to enthusiasm. If your presentation requires a microphone, use it, rather than eyeing it suspiciously or moving around so that the volume of your voice changes. Giving a good presentation requires acting skills. Dress conservatively, smartly and comfortably. People should not be distracted by what you are wearing.

The authors have experienced being videoed giving presentations and then critiqued by a professional presenter. Often people have habits that they are not even aware of – one of ours was hand wringing. Box 27.1 has some tips on body language.

In terms of the content of your presentation, make sure it is clear, well structured with a beginning, middle and end. Start by setting the scene and

---

Box 27.1 Body language

- Stand still with both feet apart and one foot slightly forward
- Use a lectern for security and notes
- Put your arms by your sides or on the lectern apart from the occasional gesture
- Face the audience
- Make eye contact with all areas of the room
- Smile
- Be enthusiastic
- Be natural
- Know your bad habits, for example covering your mouth when speaking, making funny faces, scratching your nose, nervous cough, etc.

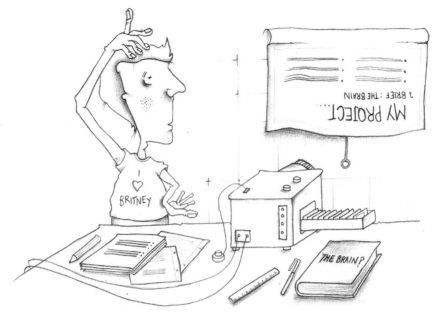

Presentations.

motivating the audience that their valuable time is going to be well spent. Use humour carefully and make sure it fits the subject matter. Appropriate questions (whether rhetorical, answered by you or the audience) can get people thinking. Try to use graphs, pictures, stories or examples to illustrate what you are saying. Keep the energy going until the very end and leave the audience with a clear message – your main point.

Death by PowerPoint

We have all attended presentations where we could not read the slides. Presentations are definitely a case of 'less is more'. Can you get your message across in less words than you intend to use? Too many pictures, fancy PowerPoint slide transitions and (worse) sound effects can also detract from the main message. Box 27.2 has some suggestions for the effective use of PowerPoint.

Always be prepared for the fact that the technology might go wrong. Check in advance whether the computer you will be using has a USB port or a CD-Rom player. For really high stakes presentations (e.g. at an interview) it is wise to have your set of slides on back-up transparencies as well. If travelling abroad, when things can get lost, post your presentation to your web mail account before setting off. This all sounds a bit paranoid but the old maxim 'if it can go wrong, it will go wrong' does apply to the interaction between humans and electronic equipment!

Box 27.2 Using PowerPoint

- Only use contrasting colours, for example white text on a dark blue background or black text on a white background
- Use no more than two colours per slide
- Do not use capital letters – they are difficult to read
- Plan your talk using roughly 1 minute per slide
- Use large font (e.g. 24–32 point)
- There should be roughly 6 bullet points per slide
- Avoid cute Clipart
- Practise using PowerPoint so you know how to get your talk on the screen.

If you are using an overhead projector, you can make your transparencies using PowerPoint. Follow the same rules above. There is nothing worse than unreadable overhead projections, especially ones that are slowly revealed by the speaker!

Workshops

At some stage in your career you may be asked to take part in or run a workshop. Workshops are learning episodes which usually last longer than a lecture, presentation or small group teaching (e.g. half a day or a day) and contain a variety of teaching methods which work towards the overall aims and objectives. For example, a session on non-invasive ventilation would be ideal as a workshop. The protected teaching afternoons that many Foundation Programme trainees and other doctors have would also be ideal in a workshop format. Workshops usually contain lectures, small group work, practical exercises (e.g. simulated scenarios) and feedback. As workshops are interactive and contain a variety of teaching methods, learning can be far more effective than sitting in a room listening to a series of lectures.

The key to running a workshop is planning. You need to ask yourself the same three questions you ask before giving a lecture (see Chapter 25). Make sure the learning objectives are realistic for the time you have and then think about how you can use different teaching methods to achieve these. An example plan for a workshop is shown in Box 27.3.

Posters

Another common way of presenting information is with a poster. Most specialist society conferences have poster sessions. Posters can be visually powerful and allow the reader time to digest information. Most hospital media services print posters. It is less expensive and quicker if you design the poster

Box 27.3 Example workshop plan

Acute care training for 5th year medical students
Objectives – by the end of the day the students will be able to:
- Recognise an acutely ill patient
- Be able to initially manage an acutely ill patient
- Be able to communicate effectively to senior colleagues about an acutely ill patient
- Understand the bigger picture regarding acute care in the National Health Service (NHS).

Workshop plan (20 students in total)

Time	Subject	
0930–1030	Lecture: recognising critical illness and the ABCDE system	
	Group 1	*Group 2*
Split in to two tutorial groups 1030–1115	Oxygen therapy	Blood gases
1115–1200	Blood gases	Oxygen therapy
All together 1200–1215	SimMan™ demonstration	
1215–1245	Lunch	
Split into two tutorial groups 1245–1415	Fluids and volume resuscitation	Simulated scenarios using SimMan™
1415–1430	Coffee break	
1430–1600	Simulated scenarios using SimMan™	Fluids and volume resuscitation
All together 1600–1620	Short lecture: summary of the ABCDE system	
1620–1630	Course evaluation	

yourself using PowerPoint and hand it to them electronically, but you can still give them a large piece of paper with bits glued to it and ask them to do the designing for you. Allow plenty of time for this.

Conference organisers usually dictate the dimensions of the poster, so make sure you know what these are before proceeding. Text should be legible at a

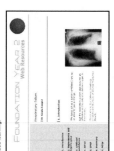
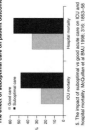
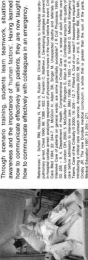

Figure 27.1 Example poster.

viewing distance of 1 m. The layout should be clear and logical and should include:
- The title
- Names and institutions of the authors
- Introduction
- Methods
- Results
- Discussion
- References.

When designing a poster, remember that 'a picture tells a thousand words' and try not to cram in a lot of text. Laptops with audio–visual displays are sometimes used alongside posters and handouts can convey more information and contact details as well. If you are at a conference with posters, wander around and make a note of which posters grab your attention and why.

Good posters attract interest and tell a story. They also:
- Grab your attention
- Are easy to read from a distance
- Encourage interaction
- Use images to convey essential information concisely.

Fig. 27.1 shows an example of a poster.

Key points: Presentations

- Presentations are for getting your message across – what is your main message?.
- Presenting is like putting on a performance, although it is important to be natural as well.
- Be careful in your use of audio–visual aids.
- Always plan a presentation or workshop with the aims and objectives in mind.
- Poster presentations are commonly used in medicine and use images as well as text to convey a message.

Exercises

- Ask an experienced presenter to watch you give a 5-minute presentation. Take only 5 minutes to prepare.
- Think about presentations that you have seen recently. What aspects did you enjoy most? What would you change about them to make them better?
- Think about protected teaching afternoons you have experienced. Are these usually in a lecture format? What are the aims and objectives of these sessions? How could they be changed to a workshop format? Would this improve your learning?
- Plan to present a poster at a conference within the next 12 months. This could be an audit project you have completed, for example.

Reference

1. Mehrabian A. *Silent Messages: Implicit Communication of Emotions and Attitudes*, 2nd edn. Wadsworth, Belmont, CA, 1981.

Further resources

- Dixon B. Sorry, you won't be able to see this... *BMJ* 1996; **313**: 1407.
- Newble D and Cannon R. Making a presentation at a conference. In: *A Handbook for Medical Teachers*, 4th edn. Kluwer Academic Publishers, Dordrecht, 2001.

CHAPTER 28

Teaching a skill

By the end of this chapter you will be able to:

- Describe the learning curve
- Plan how to teach a practical skill
- Know how to use the 4-step approach to teaching a practical skill
- Know how to supervise someone learning a practical procedure

Teaching a practical skill is different to other forms of teaching. At some point the learner has to perform the procedure on a patient and, by definition, they are not yet skilled in carrying out the task. Patient safety therefore is a more immediate issue compared with learning how to take a history or make a diagnosis.

Doctors all have to monitor and teach skills, whether this is teaching medical students how to insert an intravenous cannula, Senior House Officers (SHOs) about ultrasound guided central venous access or senior doctors a new laparoscopic technique.

Learning curves

It takes many repetitions of a skill to become proficient at it. There is no predetermined number of times that it should be performed and trainees often vary in the rate at which they achieve proficiency. When starting to learn a procedure, the success rate is often low. There is usually a rapid improvement over the first 20 or so procedures, with further improvement over the next 100 [1]. A method that allows success rate to be easily plotted has been described by Kestin [2].

Without supervision, learners show a higher complication rate than experienced practitioners. However with appropriate supervision, the complication rate amongst learners remains comparable to that seen in the hands of an experienced person [3]. The key to maintaining patient safety is therefore proper supervision, so that the learner can learn, whilst the patient remains safe.

Research has shown that confidence and competence are not the same thing. When trainees are rated on their confidence in performing a practical procedure and then observed doing so, the two do not correlate [4].

Teaching a practical skill does require some planning. The stages that need to be considered are: preparation, performing the procedure and review.

Preparation

Several elements are essential in order for a teacher to teach a practical skill. The teacher must be sufficiently familiar with the technique and potential complications that he is able to anticipate difficulties and retrieve any situation. He must be able to perform the skill automatically in order to be able to direct his attention to teaching. The teacher must have sufficient authority to be accepted as a master by the learner. He must be able to stop the learner from continuing if there are concerns about patient safety.

It takes time to teach a practical procedure and it is unrealistic to expect that the procedure can be taught in the same time that it takes a proficient operator to perform the task. It is essential to ensure that time is available and to forewarn any others who may be affected by any delay. Failing to create the extra time required places unnecessary pressure on both the learner and the teacher. Patients may then suffer as a result. You should also ensure that the patient is not too difficult a case on which to learn.

Beforehand, the teacher should discuss the procedure with the trainee and define exactly what it is he is expected to do. Does the trainee understand the indications, complications and relevant anatomy for this procedure? Does he understand how to judge the success or failure of the task? Apparently simple procedures actually contain a number of steps which are required in order to be successful (see Box 28.1). A good teacher needs to be able to break a procedure down in this way.

Performing the procedure

Adopting a 4-step approach is a useful way to teach a practical skill. You may be familiar with this approach from advanced life support (ALS) or advanced trauma life support (ATLS) courses:

- *Step 1*: Demonstrate the procedure at normal speed. The learner becomes more aware of what the skill involves.
- *Step 2*: Demonstrate the procedure with explanations and questions. It is important to emphasise what you are doing and why. This will not be apparent from just watching what you are doing. For instance, if inserting an intravenous cannula, an observer will not know why you decided to give up on one site and attempt another simply from watching.
- *Step 3*: Repeat the procedure and get the trainee to describe each step this time. Here you are able to check that the learner has understood the main points before they perform the task on a patient.
- *Step 4*: The trainee does and describes each step themselves. They are telling you what they are doing, whilst they are doing it.

Box 28.1 The steps in inserting an intravenous cannula

- Choose cannula size
- Assemble necessary equipment
- Discuss with patient
- Place tourniquet on arm
- Ask patient to make fist
- Choose appropriate vein
- Sterilise skin
- Stretch skin until taught
- Pierce skin with needle
- Direct cannula into vein until see flashback
- Withdraw needle until tip rests within cannula sheath
- Direct cannula along direction of vein
- Remove tourniquet
- Occlude end of cannula within vein/raise limb to prevent bleeding when needle withdrawn
- Remove needle
- Place cap on end of cannula
- Discard needle into sharps bin
- Secure cannula
- Draw up saline flush
- Flush cannula.

Only some of these steps are obvious from pure observation. Many of the steps will require some explanation for the observer to fully appreciate what each step involves.

The benefit of this approach is that you as supervisor know what the learner is about to do before they actually perform it for real on a patient. This is particularly important as an awake patient will not be reassured by you giving step-by-step instructions.

It can sometimes be difficult to adopt this approach, as it takes four repetitions of the task before the learner has reached step 4. Part-task simulators and clinical skills labs can be invaluable when a learner is totally unfamiliar with a skill.

Some practical skills are actually quite complicated. In these cases it can be beneficial to break down the task into sections, and get the learner to concentrate on becoming familiar with one step before he moves on to the next. This is less overwhelming. Try not to distract the learner by talking to them or questioning them whilst they are performing the task. It requires intense concentration for them to carry out a task they have only just become accustomed to.

Review

Review and feedback is important in moving the learner on to the next stage by reinforcing good practice and highlighting areas to concentrate on next time. Review following a practical procedure should follow the principles of feedback discussed in Chapter 29:
- Ask, 'What do you think went well?' followed by what you think went well.
- Ask, 'What could you have done differently/do differently next time?' followed by what you think about this.
- If you have concerns, ask 'What do you think of the way you did...?'
- Emphasise correct performance rather than what was done badly.
- Check to ensure that the learner has understood the feedback.
- Agree an action plan if needed.

Supervising movement along the learning curve

A different approach is needed in order to supervise someone who has already reached some degree of independence. This entails finding out what the learner knows already. You need to find out what the learner is planning to do before they do it. This also gives you the opportunity to find out which areas they find difficult, in order to concentrate your teaching on that area. The following questions are useful:
- How many have you done?
- How long ago?
- With what degree of success?
- What bits do you find easy?
- What bits do you find harder?
- Tell me about the last time it did not work as intended.
- Tell me what you are going to do when you do this procedure.
- How will you know when to stop and let me take over?

This series of questions allows you to gauge the learner's experience and knowledge of the procedure and identify areas which may be causing difficulty. The last question is important, as it allows you to set some clear and explicit ground rules as to when the learner will hand the procedure over to you. This allows you to intervene without unduly worrying the patient. You should be wary of teaching anyone who is unable to answer the above questions.

Performing a practical procedure is more than just a technical skill. Whilst correct technical performance is essential, this is of little value if the procedure has been performed on a patient in whom it was not warranted in the first place. All practical procedures require underpinning knowledge and attitudes as well.

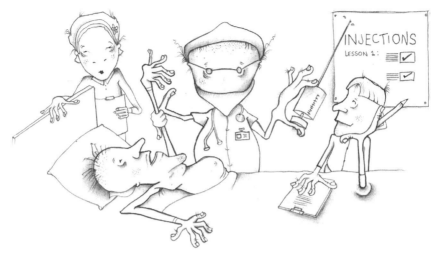

Teaching a skill.

Key points: Teaching a skill

- Patient safety should always be the first concern when teaching a practical skill.
- Ensure you have time to teach a skill properly.
- A learner's confidence and competence are not the same thing.
- The stages of teaching a practical skill are: preparation, performing the procedure and review.
- Find out what the learner is going to do before he does it.
- Performing a practical procedure is more than just a technical skill.

Exercises

- You are asked to teach some medical students how to examine the respiratory system. Devise a lesson plan involving the 4-step approach.
- Think of a practical procedure in which you are competent and try and break it down in to its constituent steps.
- Have you experienced a situation in which confidence and competence were not the same thing? What happened?
- Do you take responsibility for learning the theory behind common practical procedures (e.g. the maximum safe dose of lignocaine)?

References

1. Prasad S. Phaco-emulsification learning curve. *Journal of Cataract and Refractive Surgery* 1998; **24**: 73–77.

2. Kestin IG. A statistical approach to measuring the competence of anaesthetic trainees at practical procedures. *British Journal of Anaesthesiology* 1995; **75**: 805–809.
3. Titley OG and Bracka A. A 5 year audit of trainees experience and outcomes with two-stage hypospadias surgery. *British Journal of Plastic Surgery* 1998; **51**: 370–375.
4. Barnsley L, Lyon PM, Ralston SJ *et al.* Clinical skills in junior medical officers: a comparison of self-reported confidence and observed competence. *Medical Education* 2004; **38**: 358–367.

CHAPTER 29

How to give feedback

By the end of this chapter you will be able to:

- Know the components of effective feedback
- Understand the reasons for poor feedback
- Be able to follow a model of providing effective feedback
- Know how to receive feedback

One of the keys to learning is feedback. Experience without feedback is educationally meaningless. Feedback helps us to stay on the right track and motivates us to continue learning. The medical profession has traditionally not been very good at providing educationally useful feedback. Surveys of trainees find that stress and depression are common and that positive feedback is rarely given [1].

It has long been recognised that learning and performance can be vastly improved with constructive (rather than destructive) feedback. Since all doctors are teachers, all doctors need to learn how to give as well as receive feedback.

Think of a time when you were given feedback, for example on a post-take ward round, after dealing with an emergency, performing a procedure or discussing a case in clinic. What did that feedback consist of? How did you receive it? Sometimes feedback does not work and there are many reasons why this might be. These include:

- Most teachers have not been taught how to give effective feedback.
- People tend to give feedback only when something goes wrong.
- Feedback may be taken personally and this puts people off giving and receiving it.
- The teacher or educational supervisor may not have observed your performance enough to give feedback.
- Learners may not recognise when feedback *is* being given.

Research in medical education has looked at what makes feedback educationally effective. The idea of feedback is that it will result in a change in knowledge, skills or attitudes. Studies have highlighted the need for 'interactive' feedback. This includes self-assessment by the trainee, allowing the trainee to react to the feedback provided and an action plan which the trainee develops under guidance. It is effective feedback, rather than the assessment itself, which promotes growth in the trainee's clinical skills.

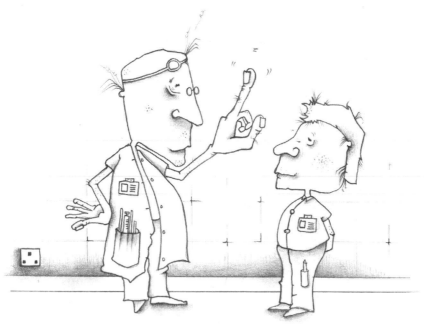

Feedback.

Effective feedback is:
- Based on knowledge of actual performance rather than hearsay
- Constructive
- Timely (close in time to the observed event)
- Specific rather than general (based on facts rather than impressions)
- Consistent (not conflicting with previous information)
- Face to face
- Received (sometimes it is not the right time – ask the other person if you can give feedback).

For example, comments such as, "Communication with colleagues appears to be a problem" without giving an example is not very helpful. Whereas, "When you spoke with sister yesterday you appeared very angry" could form the basis of a constructive conversation.

Principles of feedback

The basic principles of feedback can be divided into three areas: setting the stage, timing, and the actual content. These are summarised as follows:

Setting the stage
- Establish a relationship with the learner that emphasises working together with common goals.

- Create an environment of trust, where learners welcome constructive feedback.
- Ensure that goals and/or objectives are clearly understood by both the person giving feedback and the learner.
- For feedback that may be construed as negative, find a quiet, private, comfortable place.

Timing
- Make feedback a regular occurrence
- Feedback should be as immediate as possible.

Content
- Use the 'feedback sandwich' – start with positive things, then specify areas that need improvement, then end on an encouraging note.
- Learners should have the opportunity to assess their own performance first. "What do you think went well?" is a good place to start. This should be followed with, "What could you have done differently?" and finally an action plan to improve performance.
- Use descriptive, non-pejorative language that focuses on actions rather than an individual's abilities or character.
- Emphasise correct performance rather than what was done badly.
- Limit the quantity of feedback given at any one time.
- Check to ensure that the learner has understood the feedback.
- Follow up on the agreed action plan.

The feedback sandwich is not just a 'touchy-feely' way of giving feedback. It is used in order to make feedback more effective. Feedback is only educationally useful if the learner does something with it. Starting with positive points shows you paid attention, demonstrates empathy towards someone who is learning and makes people more likely to take on board what you have to say. This is particularly important if you do not know the person.

The reason why learners should have the opportunity to comment on their own performance first is because many do have insight into their own performance. As a teacher you can reassure and encourage their own self-assessment. Using this method also forewarns you if the learner lacks insight. Poorly performing doctors tend to over-rate themselves whereas good doctors tend to under-rate themselves.

An action plan may be something as simple as reading guidelines on the management of a condition, or the teacher could help the trainee spend time in another department in order to practise a skill.

Do not try to correct everything at once. Even if there is a long list of things that went wrong, only discuss one or two (maximum three) and be specific. The trainee will not remember any more detail than this and his motivation will wane. Teachers should help learners take small steps, using periodic mini-evaluations to summarise their overall performance and design specific learning activities based on their assessment and feedback.

Very occasionally a doctor's performance may be so poor as to be a danger to patients. It may then be appropriate to restrict that doctor's activities. If this happens, it should be accompanied by clear and transparent communication in which all parties identify the problems and agree on an appropriate action plan to remedy these.

Receiving feedback

We all need to learn how to receive constructive feedback when it is given, as many of us have little insight into some of our behaviours; 360° feedback is a formal method of feedback in which most doctors now participate. The following are tips on how to receive constructive feedback:

- Listen actively
- Try to understand this is not an attack on your character
- Ask questions to make sure you understand what is being said
- Understand that other people see things differently and have different experience
- Even if you do not agree with everything that is being said, there will be some good ideas for you to think about and work on
- Devote your energy to improving your performance rather than disputing someone else's observations
- Engage in the process and offer ideas of your own.

Some people are not very good at giving feedback. Sometimes it is best to simply realise this and learn how not to give feedback yourself!

Key points: Feedback

- Effective feedback is essential for learning.
- Feedback should be constructive, timely, specific and consistent.
- Feedback should be interactive, covering positive things first then areas needing improvement.
- Feedback may require an action plan and follow-up.
- Be able to receive and act on feedback yourself.

Exercises

- Discuss your experiences of destructive feedback, either to yourself or others. What effect did this feedback have? What are the features of destructive feedback?
- Discuss a time when you received feedback that was helpful to you. What were the things about it that made it helpful?
- How often do you give praise when it is due?
- How often do you give constructive feedback when you observe a colleague who needs to improve his performance?
- In a group of two practice giving and receiving feedback following the steps above. Remember it is the person who is receiving the feedback who starts by reflecting on his own performance.

Reference

1. Luck C. Reducing stress among junior doctors. *Student BMJ* 2001; **9**: 16–17.

Further resource

• Mets B. Giving feedback and monitoring progress. In: Greaves *et al.*, eds. *Clinical Teaching – A Guide to Teaching Practical Anaesthesia*. Swets and Zeitlinger Publishers, Lisse, The Netherlands, 2003.

CHAPTER 30
How doctors are assessed

By the end of this chapter you will be able to:

• Understand the different assessment methods used in Foundation Programmes
• Know about the continuing assessment of all doctors
• Know the key organisations relating to doctors in training

Over the last decade there have been many changes to the way doctors are trained, ranging from changes to the undergraduate curriculum, specialist training, working hours and more recently 'Modernising Medical Careers' (MMC) [1] which aims to introduce shorter, more structured, competency-based postgraduate medical education. Every new medical graduate in the UK enters a 2-year Foundation Programme [2] which has two educational themes: generic skills (the subject of this book) and acute care (the subject of our companion book) [3]. The aim is that every new doctor in the UK should be competent in the following broad areas:
• Clinical and communication skills
• Legal and ethical issues
• Patient safety
• Teaching and learning
• The recognition and management of an acutely ill patient.
To facilitate this learning, work-based assessments have been introduced. These are designed to help good doctors improve by providing an opportunity for structured feedback. They are also designed to identify the minority of doctors who are underperforming and need remedial training. To move beyond the Foundation Programme, a doctor has to demonstrate competence by having a series of satisfactory assessments which cover a range of knowledge, skills and attitudes.

In England and Wales, the work-based assessments are:
• Mini-CEX (clinical evaluation exercise)
• DOPS (direct observation of procedural skills)
• 360° feedback: mini-PAT (peer assessment tool) or TAB (team assessment of behaviour)
• CBD (case-based discussion).
The assessments in Foundation Programmes are designed to be part of a normal working day. Their validity, reliability and feasibility have been studied.

Medical students demonstrate their knowledge by multiple choice questions (MCQs) and that they know *how* to do something by objective structured clinical examinations (OSCEs). Work-based assessments assess actual performance (see Miller's pyramid in Chapter 24). A number of studies have shown that new graduates are not competent in a range of clinical skills, despite having passed finals [4].

Mini-CEX

The mini-CEX is a short observed clinical encounter. An ideal setting for this is in the Accident and Emergency department, during a post-take ward round or during a clinic or home visit. The focus of the mini-CEX in Foundation Programmes is acute care.

A patient encounter consists of three parts: interview, examination and counselling. The mini-CEX should take only one of these (approximately 15 minutes) and then spend around 5 minutes on feedback. Examples of mini-CEX opportunities include:
- Taking a history for collapse ?cause
- Examination of the abdomen
- Obtaining informed consent for a procedure
- Explaining a diagnosis and management plan
- Assessing a sick patient using the ABCDE system.

A different aspect should be covered each time. Mini-CEX has been developed in US residency programmes where it has been found to be logistically feasible compared with a full CEX, yet still reliable and valid, with high satisfaction among trainees [5].

DOPS

DOPS is similar to mini-CEX except a practical procedure is being observed. A list of procedures in which Foundation trainees should demonstrate competence is listed in Box 30.1, but other procedures can be assessed as well. As many different procedures as possible should be observed.

The acquisition of expertise has the following key requirements [6]:
- Sustained deliberate practice
- Feedback
- Ongoing experience.

The assessor should be able to perform the practical skill being observed and, unless there is a threat to patient safety, leave questions and feedback to the end. Assessors can find DOPS difficult for the following reasons:
- There may not be an agreed standard for performing a procedure
- The assessors themselves may never have learned the procedure correctly
- The learning curve (described in Chapter 28)
- The level of competence expected of an F1 and F2 trainee may be unclear.

Assessor training is therefore important, and is discussed further below.

Box 30.1 Procedures that Foundation trainees should be competent and confident to perform

F1 (house officer year):
- Venepuncture and intravenous (i.v.) cannulation
- Use of local anaesthesia
- Blood cultures
- Injections (subcutaneous, intradermal, intramuscular)
- Preparation and administration of i.v. medication
- Prescribing i.v. fluids including blood
- Electrocardiogram (including interpretation)
- Spirometry (including interpretation)
- Urethral catheterisation
- Basic airway management
- Nasogastric tube insertion.

F2 (first senior house officer year) – speciality specific procedures, for example:
- Aspiration of pleural fluid or air
- Skin suturing
- Lumbar puncture
- Insertion of central venous cannula
- Aspiration of a large joint.

Training in practical procedures should include study of the theory as well as practical observation and experience.

360° feedback

360° (or multi-source) feedback mainly assesses competency in the knowledge, skills and attitudes listed in 'Good Medical Practice' [7], that is, communication skills and professional behaviour. These are areas in which problems and complaints most frequently occur. A minimum number of raters across a specified range of professions is needed to make the assessment reliable and this holds true even when the trainee chooses the individual raters [8].

360° feedback is particularly valuable for providing individualised feedback to doctors about important non-clinical skills such as:
- Relationships with patients
- Communication with colleagues
- Accessibility and reliability
- Ability to prioritise
- Willingness to teach.

CBD

Case-based discussion can focus on acute care or generic skills and is designed to be a 10–15-minute discussion of a case, using the medical record made by

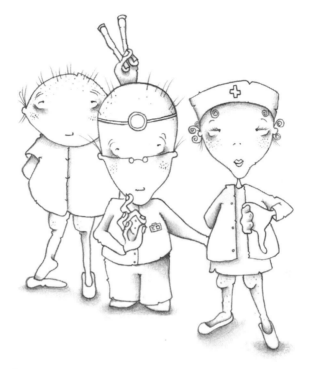

360° feedback.

the trainee at the time. As with the other assessments, a minimum number of cases with as many different assessors as possible is required to ensure good reliability.

For example, a case of a patient in pain could be used to discuss the analgesic ladder or an ethical situation could be explored. CBD is not an opportunity to discuss other people's management of the case, nor is it a viva on medical facts unrelated to the entry made by the trainee. It is designed to explore the trainee's understanding and thought processes and provide an opportunity for feedback, reflection and learning.

In a 10–15-minute discussion only two or three dimensions can be covered (e.g. medical record keeping, investigations and treatment) and each assessor should try and cover aspects which have not previously been discussed. The assessor should use open questions and allow the trainee to talk through the subject first, so that the trainee's understanding and insight can be assessed.

Training the trainers

Errors can occur in the assessment process and assessors need to be trained in order to avoid these. Training includes:
- Observation training (patient consent, how to observe, the forms themselves, practice)

- Performance dimension training (whether assessing knowledge, skills, clinical judgment or professionalism)
- Frame of reference training (the agreed standard and the acceptable standard for F1 and F2)
- How to give effective feedback (Chapter 29).

Problems observed during research includes assessors who:

- Do not actually observe
- Are too lenient or too harsh
- Do not discriminate the performance of a trainee across different dimensions of competency
- May not possess the skills which they are observing.

To get around these problems, a minimum number of observed encounters are required to ensure reliability and as many different trained assessors as possible are required to ensure validity. For example, a trainee should not have the same person observe him doing all of his mini-CEXs. Structured rating forms are used.

If a trainee performs poorly on an assessment, there should be opportunity for feedback and an action plan before re-assessment. Only the satisfactory assessments need to be submitted to the central administrative centre.

As one researcher put it, 'The major challenge that lies ahead for medical educators is how to ensure that the educators themselves possess strong clinical skills but also have the necessary skill to effectively observe, evaluate and provide feedback to trainees [9]'. Training educational supervisors and assessors is a key challenge for any local Foundation Programme, for without it observations may be prone to error and the entire assessment process lack educational value.

The continuing assessment of all doctors

All doctors are now regularly assessed during training and as a general practitioner (GP), consultant or non-consultant career grade. The Royal Colleges are developing work-based assessments for doctors after Foundation Programmes (e.g. mini-CEX, DOPS, 360° feedback and exit examinations in some specialities).

Senior doctors are regularly assessed by:

- Keeping a record of continuing professional development
- Annual appraisal
- Work-based assessments (e.g. 360° feedback)
- Revalidation every 5 years.

Appraisal is a contractual requirement for all non-trainee doctors in the National Health Service (NHS). Although appraisal is not the same as assessment, appraisal is nevertheless used in the revalidation process. Appraisal is designed to:

- Provide supportive feedback
- Recognise an individual's contribution
- Balance support with challenge to help the individual develop.

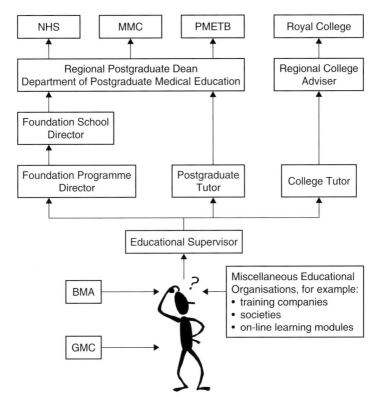

Figure 30.1 Key organisations involved in a doctor's training.

During an appraisal meeting, the doctor will meet with a trained colleague and have a discussion based around the seven core headings in 'Good Medical Practice [7]'. These are:
• Good clinical care
• Maintaining good medical practice
• Teaching and training
• Working with colleagues
• Relationships with patients
• Probity
• Health.

The appraisal discussion requires evidence relevant to the doctor's clinical practice, for example 360° feedback reports, complaints data, continuing professional development, etc. [10].

Outside bodies

The key organisations which affect doctors in training in the UK (see Fig.30.1) are:
• General Medical Council (GMC)
• Postgraduate Deaneries

- Royal Colleges
- Postgraduate Medical Education and Training Board (PMETB)
- The British Medical Association (BMA)
- Medical defence organisations.

The GMC

The GMC is the regulatory body of the medical profession and all doctors must be registered with it in order to work. The GMC carries out its role by 'keeping an up-to-date register of qualified doctors, fostering good medical practice, promoting high standards of medical education, and dealing firmly and fairly with doctors whose fitness to practise is in doubt'. The GMC regulates medical schools and the first postgraduate year (F1) in the UK by inspection against agreed standards as described in Tomorrow's Doctors [11]. Full registration is granted after satisfactory completion of F1. A comprehensive review of under-graduate medical education was launched in 2005, including consideration of a national examination for all medical students.

The GMC recognises 1600 primary medical qualifications throughout the world. Non-European Union graduates can apply for registration with the GMC by demonstrating they are capable to practice in the UK, usually by passing the Professional and Linguistic Assessment Board (PLAB) examination.

The GMC does not set standards for postgraduate training after the F1 year. This is the responsibility of the PMETB.

Postgraduate Deaneries

The Postgraduate Deaneries are part of the NHS and are responsible for ensuring the delivery of appropriate training for doctors and dentists in their geographical area. The Dean of postgraduate medical education works closely with Royal College advisers. Deaneries have to balance and plan for the training needs of doctors as well as the service requirements of the NHS. Deaneries co-ordinate the employment of Foundation doctors across the UK through MDAP (multi-deanery appointment process).

The Dean of postgraduate medical education is responsible for:
- Approving posts that are suitable for training
- Inspecting Trusts to ensure an appropriate educational environment for doctors in training
- Distributing national training numbers (NTNs or specialist registrar (SpR) posts)
- Contributing to regional and national policy on medical education and workforce planning
- Being a focal point for information and advice on postgraduate medical education and workforce planning
- Developing medical education as a speciality
- Liaising with Universities, Royal Colleges, PMETB, the NHS and other stakeholders
- Dealing with trainees in difficulty.

The Dean for postgraduate medical education can require an individual to enter remedial training or refer a doctor to the GMC if his or her fitness to practise is brought into question.

The Royal Colleges

The Royal Colleges set standards for basic and specialist training and continuing professional development. Colleges set national examinations which any doctor wishing to become a specialist must pass. They inspect training programmes around the country to ensure the right balance between training and service. They recommend, with the Deanery, a doctor to the PMETB for a Certificate of Completion of Training (CCT) and access to the specialist register, which allows a doctor to become an independent practitioner in that speciality. In addition, colleges work to improve the standards of professional practice in their speciality. They lobby governments to pursue improvements in their field through public health measures, public awareness and better funding.

Postgraduate Medical Education and Training Board

The PMETB came into existence by law in September 2005. Its principle role is 'establishing standards and requirements for postgraduate medical education and training, making sure these standards and requirements are met and developing and promoting postgraduate medical education and training across the country [12]'. It is a supervisory body, working with the Deaneries and Colleges. Its role is to evaluate training and assessment programmes and the PMETB now regulates all medical training from the second Foundation year to CCT.

The BMA

The BMA is the main professional association for doctors and membership is voluntary. It is the voice of doctors and medical students working in the UK. It advises individual doctors and represents the collective interests of the medical profession. The various roles that the BMA serve include:
- Representing the view of doctors to the media
- Publishing medical news bulletins
- Lobbying the government on health issues
- Negotiating doctors' pay and pension deals at a national level
- Providing a counselling service for sick or stressed doctors
- Providing ethical guidance to the medical profession
- Helping refugee doctors
- Lobbying the Department of Health on issues relating to various groups of doctors (e.g. non-consultant career grades)
- Providing educational and library services
- Provide individual support and advice to doctors in dispute with their employer (e.g. conditions of employment, rotas, contract, salary or disciplinary problems).

Medical defence organisations

Medical defence organisations [13] provide professional indemnity policies and legal advice. All doctors should join a medical defence organisation since Trusts do not cover doctors for acts which take place outside work (e.g. good Samaritan acts or working abroad) nor criminal proceedings. Medical defence organisations provide individual legal advice, represent you if you are sued personally and can coach you through legal or disciplinary proceedings, for example a Court appearance. They also provide a valuable educational service, helping doctors to reduce risk and complaints and provide a telephone service for advice on ethical or legal matters.

Key points: How doctors are assessed

- MMC aims to introduce shorter, more structured, competency-based postgraduate medical education.
- Foundation Programmes have two main educational themes: generic skills and acute care.
- The assessments used in the Foundation Programmes and beyond are designed to assess actual performance in the workplace.
- Assessors need to be trained to effectively observe, evaluate and provide feedback to trainees.
- GPs, consultants and non-consultant career grades have to take part in annual appraisal.
- There are several outside organisations which affect doctors in training in the UK.

Exercises

- Discuss your experiences of work-based assessments. Were your assessors trained in the assessment methods used?
- Do you understand the difference between the BMA, Deaneries and Royal Colleges?

References

1. Modernising Medical Careers in England www.mmc.nhs.uk, in Scotland www.mmc.scot.nhs.uk/Foundation_Programme, in Wales www.cardiff.ac.uk/pgmde/hospital_practice/modernising_medical_careers, in Northern Ireland www.nimdta.gov.uk
2. Curriculum for the foundation years in postgraduate education and training. www.mmc.nhs.uk/pages/foundation/Curriculum
3. Cooper N, Forrest K and Cramp P. *Essential Guide to Acute Care*, 2nd edn. Blackwells, Oxford, 2006.
4. Fox RA, Clark CLI, Scotland AD and Dacre JE. A study of pre-registration house officers' clinical skills. *Medical Education* 2000; **34**: 1007–1012.

5. Kogan JR, Bellini LM and Shea JA. Feasibility, reliability and validity of the mini-clinical evaluation exercise in a medicine core clerkship. *Academic Medicine* 2003; **78(10) Suppl**: S33–S35.
6. Kneebone RL, Nestel D, Moorthy K *et al.* Learning the skills of flexible sigmoidoscopy – the wider perspective. *Medical Education* 2003; **37 Suppl 1**: 50–58.
7. General Medical Council. Good Medical Practice, 2001. www.gmc-uk.org/guidance/good_medical_practice/index.asp
8. Archer JC, Norcini J and Davies H. Use of SPRAT for peer review of paediatricians in training. *British Medical Journal* 2005; **330**: 1251–1253.
9. Holmboe ES. Faculty and observation of trainees' clinical skills: problems and opportunities. *Academic Medicine* 2004; **79(1)**: 16–22.
10. Royal College of Physicians of London. Consultant appraisal in the NHS. Guidance for appraisees and appraisers. RCP, London, 2002. www.rcplondon.ac.uk/members/library/books/ConsultantAppraisal.pdf
11. General Medical Council. Tomorrow's Doctors, 2003. www.gmc-uk.org/education/undergraduate/tomorrows_doctors.asp
12. Postgraduate Medical Education and Training Board. www.pmetb.org.uk
13. Medical Defence Union www.the-mdu.com, Medical and Dental Defence Union of Scotland www.mddus.com, Medical Protection Society www.mps.org.uk

Further resources

• Norcini JJ, Blank LL, Duffy FD and Fortna G. The mini-CEX: a method for assessing clinical skills. *Annals of Internal Medicine* 2003; **138**: 476–481.
• The Foundation Programme assessments. Modernising Medical Careers. www.mmc.nhs.uk/pages/assessment (includes training videos).

Index

Note: Italicised page numbers refer to figures and tables.